Why Nude?

Thoughts and reflections on social nudity

Published by RFI Technical Services

http://pub.rfi.net

Cover art/model Flora by Adrian Anderson

http://www.adrianandersonphotography.com

ISBN: 9-780-9572432-3-1

Why Nude?

Thoughts and reflections on social nudity

by

Howard Anderson

Never have I felt more alive. The sun is sinking over a Mediterranean ruffled only by my fellow bathers. Couples roam the water's edge aware of little but themselves, parents watch their children playing in the sand or larking in the water, still more sit and relish the air of calm. We are on our first holiday as a couple again after the children have left home, my wife smiles at me in the warm French air. Swimming around lazily, I have the time to reflect on this most peaceful of scenes. Everyone is naked.

This work is about being nude in a social setting. I hope to show why people choose to live at least part of their lives without clothes, that doing so is very enjoyable and that it offers a number of valuable benefits. I am not trying to convert readers to the naturist lifestyle, the goal is freedom from pressure to conform not a shift to a different pressure.

It is not an academic work with full supporting evidence but I have tried to be as objective as possible, including arguments both for and against social nudity and to include references where appropriate.

In the enlightened world that celebrates diversity I do not think it is too much to ask to have complete freedom of dress for reasons of religion, culture and personal belief; governments and the police have no place in defining dress.

Introduction

"To be nobody but yourself in a world which is doing its best, night and day, to make you everybody else means to fight the hardest battle which any human being can fight; and never stop fighting. ". E. E. Cummings

There seems to be a strong desire on the part of many people to categorise other people. In this respect, others would describe me as a naturist or a nudist but this does not tell the truth. I enjoy the feeling of being without clothes but apart from that, I am just a human. I do not follow any "ism", I am not an "ist". Describing me or anyone else as a naturist conjures up a set of learned assumptions which immediately reduces understanding. To many, a naturist or a nudist is someone who belongs to a "nudist colony", is a strict vegetarian who tries to "go back to nature" but I am none of these. As internet writer Robert Tedder says, *"For me to regard myself as a nudist, I would also have to be a breathist, walkist, eatist, blue-eyesist, for while a motorist is someone who does driving, being without clothes is not something I do. It is my supposed natural state."* [1] For sheer convenience, the term naturist will have to do, it is the best we have. In the USA they usually use the term nudist but I make no distinction between the two words. Some argue at length over these terms but there is no common ground between them so I treat their distinctions as sterile, leading nowhere; language is not owned by groups or experts, it just happens. Similar arguments are made over the distinction between nude and naked but I treat them as synonymous.

The path I have chosen is not always easy, as Rudyard Kipling wrote, *"The individual has always had to struggle to keep from being overwhelmed by the tribe. To be your own man is a hard business. If you try it, you will be lonely often, and sometimes frightened. But no price is too high to pay for the privilege of owning yourself."*

My underlying assumption is that there cannot be anything fundamentally wrong or immoral with nudity, we were born nude. Any wrong that does exist comes from social values derived directly from religious teachings. Alfred North Whitehead put it like this: *"What is morality in any given time or place? It is what the majority then and there happen to like and immorality is what they dislike."* [2]

In western culture, apart from a small minority of religious sects or cultures, nudity is considered fine in private for live human beings and fine in public as sculpture or paintings. The problem, if there is one, lies with nudity in a social setting, being seen naked by others, possibly even by strangers, so it is the reaction of others that is feared by the nude, whether it be ridicule being ostrisized, the attention of the police or even violence. That a few find nudity something to *fear* is really very odd indeed.

In preparing this work I have tried to be as objective as possible, including arguments both for and against social nudity. It would be easy for detractors to make the allegation of confirmation bias, the willingness on the part of a proponent to accept supporting evidence as true or useful and counter evidence as unreliable. I am aware I may be accused of taking sides, that I have written this from a naturist's point of view which cannot therefore be impartial. Whilst it is true I have written it from that viewpoint, in mitigation, my researches have made me keenly aware of attitudes and feelings concerning nudity both for and against. I have taken the time and trouble to discuss them with family, friends and acquaintances and to research the attitudes to nudity found in many different spheres. I have also recognised the drawbacks of social nudity, those times and places where it is not appropriate and have reported some disturbing aspects in the history if naturism. I have tried to present the subject of social nudity using evidence not simply belief.

This is no project that once finished will be filed and forgotten only to move onto the next one. It is my life.

Why nude?

Why go naked?

That is the easy bit, it feels wonderful.

Being naked, especially in the open air or in the water, provides a marvellous feeling of freedom, of pleasure, the joy of simply being alive. It is difficult to describe in words, it is best experienced, but so many pre-conceived ideas and fears stop people from having that experience so they will never know. Such a shame.

Imagine this: after a long day, you arrive home hot and tired. After a cool drink, you enjoy the feeling of a good shower, many people do. You enjoy it not just because it gets you clean, it also feels good, it is refreshing, there is a sensual element and it is relaxing. If you recognise what I mean, you are just a short step from naturism, this is what it is all about, feeling good. Being naked around the house, the garden or on the beach simply prolongs the pleasant feeling.Here are some classic reasons why people go naked:

• It reduces stress. This cannot be easily measured but it is reported by the great majority

• You feel a significant gain in self-confidence, especially those who do not consider themselves one of the *"beautiful people"*

• It encourages a more open attitude to bodies

• It reduces feelings of body shame or guilt

• It reduces the need to rely on status symbols to bolster self esteem

• It provides a feeling of freedom out of proportion with simply discarding a few clothes

My aim all along is not to promote universal nudity but to encourage others to look upon nudity as a non-issue: *"One can argue that, just as we did not cease to be animals simply because we learned to make fire and tools, so we have never stopped being natural. Perhaps our nature as creatures includes building cities and computers, living in enormous clusters and donning complex costumes during times of social inter-change. If so, then it seems no more or less natural to dress up in a ball gown or tuxedo than to decide to spend some time in social environments where only the costume of skin is worn."* [56] A. D. Coleman

Those who have not experienced a socially nude environment have no basis for comparison, no experience with which to contrast their always dressed life. If they do try it then find it is not to their liking, that is fine, but at least they then know and do not assume. Claiming you know something without evidence to support it results in some inexplicable beliefs. *"The earth must be flat or we would fall off"*. Experience and evidence are what is needed to arrive at a sensible world. Mark Twain saw this was true. In Letters from the Earth, he wrote *"Adam and Eve entered the world naked and unashamed - naked and pure-minded. And no descendant of theirs has ever entered it otherwise. All have entered it naked, unashamed, and clean in mind. They entered it modest. They had to acquire immodesty in the soiled mind, there was no other way to get it. ... The convention mis-called "modesty" has no standard, and cannot have one, because it is opposed to nature and reason and is therefore an artificiality and subject to anyone's whim - anyone's diseased caprice."*

Mindfulness

Mindfulness is about knowing, moment by moment, what is happening to us both inside and outside. We can lose touch with this awareness and become bound up with other thoughts and feelings and in doing so, stop noticing how they affect our lives in other ways. As Professor Mark Williams, former director of the Oxford Mindfulness Centre, says *"Mindfulness also allows us to become more aware of the stream of thoughts and feelings that we experience and to see how we can become entangled in that stream in ways that are not helpful."* He goes on, *"This lets us stand back from our thoughts and start to see their patterns. Gradually, we can train ourselves to notice when our thoughts are taking over and realise that thoughts are simply 'mental events' that do not have to control us."* [3]

By going nude, you can feel the air on your skin and a physical freedom that is best experienced rather than described. To me this is a powerful way to achieve a mindful state and hence to benefit from the relaxation and awareness that follows. Mindfulness is recommended by NICE, the National Institute for Health and Care Excellence (NICE) as a way to prevent depression.

Going nude

A very common experience, especially for those new to naturism, is *"what was all the fuss about?"* What they feared did not come to pass. No ridicule, no looks in the wrong places, just people going about their lives, nude or naked. As Caroline Walker said in a report on her first experience of a nude beach, *"As I was starting to feel more and more out of place with my clothes on than without, I just striped off and threw my clothes down. To be honest it was all a bit of an anti-climax at this point, and you start to wonder why you were making such a big fuss of it: it felt so natural and normal I just resumed the usual business of applying plenty of sun cream."* [4] Non naturists seem to focus on what they would call private parts, questions such as *"where do I look?"* crop up. In fact, in a naturist environment, one behaves as one would anywhere else, nowhere do people like being stared at, especially in countries like Britain or the USA, so people don't do it in naturist places. Being nude, genitals are visible, but so what? There is nothing special about genitals, they are no better nor worse than any other part of the body. But, were you to seek a naughty part, you will find it inside the head.

The increasing number of cities hosting the World Naked Bike Ride, the WNBR, shows very clearly the widespread public acceptance of nudity. These rides stem from demonstrations against dependency on oil; they use nudity to show the vulnerability of humans not just to oil powered traffic but as vulnerable people in a polluted world. They have now evolved to include demonstrations for better bike lanes, freedom from body shame and a host of other causes.

The London rides in June each year are seen by an estimated 50-70,000 people, the vast majority of whom cheer, clap, shout encouragement or simply smile at the riders. Most take photographs, some strip off and join in. In the years in which I have ridden I have heard just one opposing comment, the old chestnut: *"what about the children?"*

That is a key question, how should children be brought up? Should the children be brought up fearing their own bodies, brought up to have so little knowledge of other people's bodies that they fall for the false size-zero idealised body promoted by the fashion industry and be exposed to the risk of developing eating disorders and the resulting lack of self-worth? Should they be brought up to be prudish and ignorant as some religions would have them?

In 2016, the UK's national body, British Naturism, published a paper outlining the damage that is does to children by prudery and the benefits that can be had from a more open attitude towards bodies. This paper, entitled Children Deserve better, is available from the BN website http://www.bn.org.uk. A key statement in the paper is that *"We want children to be innocent, but not ignorant "*. It goes on to say *"We believe that body openness and honesty protects children from the possible harmful effects of inappropriate material. They should find out about sex and how their bodies work from good education and openness instead of glamour and pornography. Children are naturally curious and if their curiosity is not answered openly then they will seek answers anywhere they can. Blocking will not prevent them as they can usually circumvent it with a facility that adults may not believe possible."* So yes sir, what about the children. The problem for nude people is that a few vociferous objectors react in ways that are out of all proportion to simple non sexual public nudity.

When I was a child, my mother would describe the Miss World beauty contest as the *"Fat Stock Show"*. Being young I did not understand, but I now realise she was teaching me about valuing people for what they are. To her, coming second in such a contest meant much more than if someone came second in a different form of contest, for example a race. Losing a running race could be due to lack of effort, but not winning a Fat Stock prize meant one was a substandard human being.

What did this mean for the rest of us? Were we all so ugly that we must be worthless? If only the beautiful people were allowed to be seen naked in photographs or in life, it de-values the rest of us who are not so fortunate. It is also too close to the Nazi ideal, they believed in a mythical, beautiful master race, the Aryans. These were the people to rule the world, others to be subjugated to their will. Blue eyed, blond, the beautiful people except that the beauty did not extend inside their heads.

Naturism improves your self-confidence because it does not matter what shape, size, colour or race you are. It does not matter if you have scars or bits missing. What does matter is that you feel free and are accepted for what you are. To non-naturists this may seem a large claim, that removing clothes has this benefit, but removing clothes also removes most of the social clues, some would say social props, that mark out people's position in life and are often used to hide behind or create a dominance- power dressing. Some newspapers, with their circulation at stake, try to claim there is something sinister or salacious about the whole thing. Without any knowledge or understanding, they assume it is all about sex. A number of practicalities come to mind that show this is not the case. If a nude man becomes sexually aroused, his erection is quite obvious. If the whole point of social nudity was arousal, it would show! A visit to any naturist environment will provide the evidence, it simply does not happen. Those seeking sexual stimulation find they need to go elsewhere.

Simply being nude is harmless. What delineates good from bad is the intention in the mind of the doer. Apart from some of the silly attitudes sometimes perpetuated in the press, it seems the majority of people do not feel too bothered about naturism, even if they don't take part. This view is well supported by a series of surveys such as those carried out in Britain [20], Canada [5] and in the USA [6] Surveys should always be treated with some circumspection as the questions asked and how they are asked are not always well controlled, but those carried out as professionally as possible always seem to show the same result. Most people when asked specifically what they thought of naturism give a positive or neutral answer. This does not mean they would join in, but they would be happy for others to follow the lifestyle without interference.

Why go naked? To feel relaxed, comfortable and free. Imagine walking on a glorious sunny day, wild flowers in full bloom, the alluring green of the South Downs, and the pleasure of the company of likeminded people. Reason enough for many to walk in the countryside, but walking without the encumbrance of clothes enhances the experience many times over.

What stops us

Why is nudity feared?

It is clear that a few people fear nudity deeply and are vociferous in their insistence that people cover small parts of the bodies at all times in public. Such reactions stem directly from religion and the teachings of a few dominant theologians such as Jerome, Augustine of Hippo or Ignatius of Loyola. One could perhaps understand why someone may not chose to go nude themselves, but why do they wish to impose that desire on everybody on pain of being fined or imprisoned? The desire to stay dressed is fine, the real puzzle is the sheer passion shown by a few to make the rest of us conform to their beliefs.

There is no available evidence of harm from social nudity, yet they insist that their view of the world is imposed on others. Rabindranath Tagore, winner of the Nobel Prize in Literature in 1913, wrote these words about the freedom of India from British rule but the ideas are universal and apply to naturism, social nudity and to any other rational area.

Where the mind is without fear and the head is held high;

Where knowledge is free;

Where the world has not been broken up into fragments by narrow domestic walls;

Where words come out from the depth of truth;

Where tireless striving stretches its arms towards perfection:

Where the clear stream of reason has not lost its way into the dreary desert sand of dead habit;

Where the mind is lead forward by thee into ever-widening thought and action;

Into that heaven of freedom, my Father, let my country awake.

In the end reason will win but it will take a concerted effort to bring it about. Leonardo da Vinci saw this all those years ago when he wrote *"First I shall test by experiment before I proceed farther, because my intention is to consult experience first and then with reasoning show why such experience is bound to operate in such a way. And this is the true rule by which those who analyse the effects of nature must proceed; and although nature begins with the cause and ends with experience, we must follow the opposite course namely, begin with experience, and by means of it investigate the cause."*

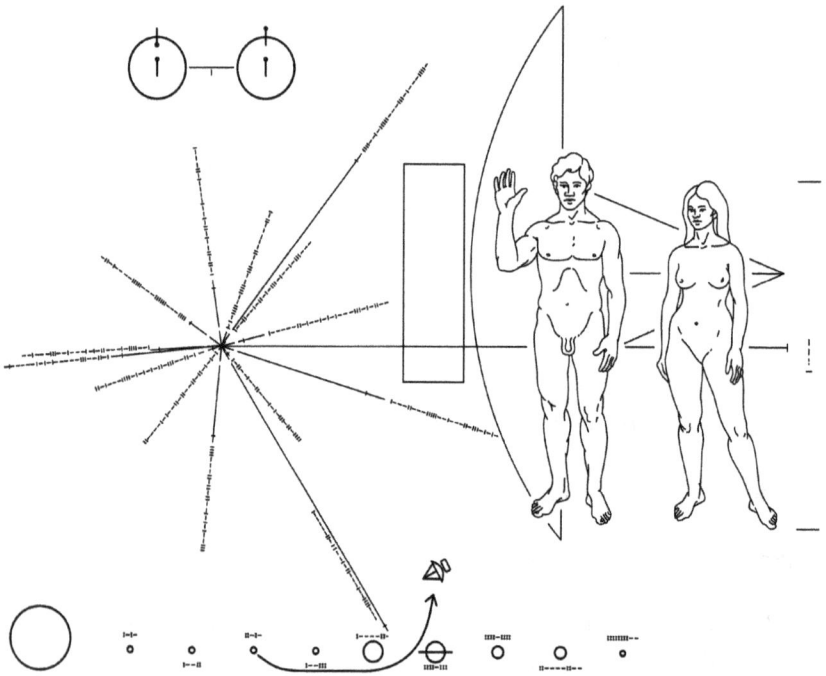

Pioneer plaque courtesy NASA/JPL-Caltech [65]

In 1972 and 1973, two of the Pioneer space missions carried a plaque in case they were ever intercepted by aliens despite there being only a vanishingly small chance of that, but it was an expression of hope and optimism. The plaques show a nude male and female in stylised form.

In 1977 the Voyager spacecraft were launched, this had more ambitious evidence of human life including music and images, but the committee that decided on its content were specifically banned from showing any nudity. This is very odd, should the craft ever be seen by alien beings then a key part of what makes us human is missing, our bodies. Did the authorities in the USA think that aliens would be corrupted by nudity? Did they think that vulnerable humans would build their own spacecraft, travel for decades through space in the hope of intercepting the craft and then be corrupted by an image of nudity? That aspect of these otherwise splendid missions is utterly absurd, but it does show the depth of irrational feelings suffered by some humans.

Why Always Stay Dressed?

There has been no evidence found in our biology to show any fundamental reason for humans to stay dressed at all times. There is the clear need to be warm, the need to be protected from the environment and the need to decorate the body and show social status but none of these provide a compelling reason to hide specific body parts in public in all circumstances and on pain of ridicule or the law.

In spite of this, there are several reasons cited for always staying dressed in a social setting, perhaps the most compelling is because everyone else does. When confronted with the possibility of going nude, perhaps on a holiday beach far from home, many people will find reasons to stay dressed even if they are attracted to the idea of feeling free. The most common reason would be embarrassment and this can be a powerful emotion. Most people are not embarrassed about body parts such as hands, feet, arms etc., so this begs the question, why are they embarrassed about their penis or their breasts? What particular aspect of these parts should lead to this feeling? Study of human behaviour shows there is no fundamental, biological reason for this, after all, naturists go naked in a social setting without detriment. Embarrassment is learned and can be unlearned. However, having once encountered a social nude environment, most people are amazed to find that their embarrassment disappears.

In addition to embarrassment, society expects us to conform. Minorities and those whose life is not widely understood are shunned and the result is much emotional pain. Kellie Maloney was born Frank Maloney and she has spent a lifetime in the very male dominated sport of boxing as a promoter. She has now come out in society as a transsexual, a process far harder than that faced by naturists, but the problems faced by each are similar in nature. Kellie writes *"It wasn't my plan to come out publicly. I was living quietly as a woman for four years before someone outed me to the press..."* The press seems to think it holds the keys to what is acceptable or not in society and that anything outside their world is ripe for exploitation, regardless of emotional damage to those outed, those who fear being outed and all their family and friends. Reports about naturists or nudists routinely use cheap pejorative language, the stock in trade of low grade hacks, these hacks seem to think it quite acceptable to hurt people and make money from doing so.

Kellie goes on, *"When people ask me if it bothers me whether my Catholic religion accepts me as a transgender person, that's what I say. I don't think religion should be used to control people."* The body shame so well represented in the press, especially the tabloids, stems directly from the Catholic Church, yet those same papers are not the voice of the church, they simply reflect old and deeply hurtful opinions- it is time they changed. The boxing promoter also says *"You wouldn't expect me or Caitlyn Jenner to be suffering from gender issues because of the very male sporting worlds we were involved in. So I do hope we'll give others the strength and courage to come out."* The very fact that that we need courage is to face an "enemy", i.e. those in the press or the clergy who have decided that they know all that is right or wrong,

12

acceptable or not, despite being often dramatically wrong themselves. If an organisation was found to be causing physical pain to those it exploited, there would be arrests, court cases and punishment, but the mob-rule nature of "moralizing" that causes so much emotional pain is not thought to be that serious. It is.

Western religions do not generally have direct prohibition of social nudity as a core belief, such prohibition as there is has come about from custom and practice and from misunderstood interpretations of early teachings. Protestations against nudity have been made by a few of the religious hierarchy and sadly followed by the many. There is often a huge difference in the core beliefs of a religion and what is taught by those who feel they should teach it. It is quite easy to find a given religious text and then to find a range of mutually opposing interpretations of that same text. A good example is the use of the word "shame" in the Christian story of Adam and Eve's expulsion from the Garden of Eden. Some Christian teachers will take it to mean that nakedness is shameful, others will take it to mean that nakedness is good; the position taken by the Christian naturist movement. How could a God have made something shameful? Would you dare suggest that the handiwork of your God is so flawed it must be covered all the time? Did He make such a serious mistake? Who are you to tell your God that He made mistakes in His creation? To me, the good or bad about nudity is what is in your heart, your intentions, the reasons you go naked, not the nudity itself.

Western women seem more reluctant to live nude. When I first started researching the subject I had the idea that the reason was because women would feel threatened or become the focus of unwanted attention, but experience shows that naturist venues feel safe and welcoming to women. It seems the real reason that women may not join in is that many fear they are not up to standard. This is an enormous shame, a symptom of the damage done by the relentless selling of the elusive image of the perfect body. The experience of millions of naturists has shown that social nudity helps to free people from a poor body image. If nothing else, experiencing social nudity shows that most people have a far from perfect body and that it does not matter a jot. A great deal of advertising in the Western world is concerned with the quest for beauty, mostly aimed at women. The implication is that if you do not spend on beauty products, you will be a lesser person, leading many women to undervalue themselves as people. Looks have nothing to do with naturism, people do not do it to be seen nor indeed to see others, they do it because it feels good. Fashion and the hunt for the perfect body only leads to dissatisfaction, this perfection is not achievable. Sadly, many women seem to feel that if they went nude, their long sought-after "look" will vanish.

Fear of sex related crime has been cited by a few as a reason they would not go naked in a social setting, but it comes as a surprise to them that there are much lower rates of sex related crime in naturist communities. Their prejudice tells them nudity must cause sexual stimulation and will therefore lead to all sorts of lewd behaviour. The experience of millions shows it doesn't. When the naturist centre at le Cap d'Agde in the South of France first opened, the local police took a close interest but experience over the years has shown this to be unnecessary. Fortunately, they are now better employed elsewhere.

Some may not go naked as a result of the opinions or reactions of others; they may be attracted to the idea but be persuaded against it. Those intent on preventing a nude lifestyle still insist that naturism is about sex although they will not have any evidence to support that view. No doubt a few people, intent on sexual gratification, will go to a naturist environment, but the sight of many less than perfect bodies does not provide their hoped for excitement and they go elsewhere. Some naturist beaches open to the public have occasional trouble from a voyeur lurking in the dunes behind the beach, but the great majority enjoy the beach in peace and for non-sexual reasons. There is plenty of evidence to support this view, the best way to collect it is to visit a large naturist resort and see for yourself. You will see people sunbathing, doing sport, walking, shopping, sailing etc., all the normal activities of holiday makers. You will not see a sex romp or any other imagined activity as would be reported in the gutter press or by religious extremists. Naturists have sex, they are no different in that respect from anyone else, but like at any holiday resort, sex is something done in private. Sadly companies in the porn industry have used the words nudist and naturist to sell their products. Those who feel the need for porn are nothing to do with naturism.

Another reason some may not consider a naturist lifestyle is worry over children. Observation shows that children are not concerned about nudity, adults are troubled in their name. Anyone who has brought up a child will know their complete lack of nudity awareness when they are little. Teaching a child to be obsessive about covering will not help them to have a healthy attitude to their body and to become a sensible well balanced adult. Perhaps this is a good place to reiterate one aim of this book, it is not to promote universal nudity, it is simply to promote the idea that nudity is as acceptable is being dressed, it is beneficial and quite quite harmless. Bringing up children is hard enough but teaching them an unnecessary layer of guilt will not help them.

The fact that an opinion has been widely held is no evidence whatever that it is not utterly absurd; indeed in view of the silliness of the majority of mankind, a widespread belief is more likely to be foolish than sensible. Bertrand Russell wrote this in his Marriage and Morals. He makes the point very well, just because always being dressed is widespread does not mean it is a Good Thing.

The most prosaic reason to stay dressed is because others do. But as Bertrand Russell wrote in his work The Conquest of Happiness, *"Conventional people are roused to fury by departure from convention, largely because they regard such departure as a criticism of themselves."*

John Lennon agreed, he wrote: *"The main hang-up in the world today is hypocrisy and insecurity. If people can't face up to the fact of other people being naked or smoking pot, or whatever they want to do, then we're never going to get anywhere. People have got to become aware that it's none of their business and that being nude is not obscene. Being ourselves is what's important. If everyone practised being themselves instead of pretending to be what they aren't, there would be peace."*

Albert Einstein followed the same idea, he wrote, *"Great spirits have always found violent opposition from mediocrities. The latter cannot understand it when a man does not thoughtlessly submit to hereditary prejudices but honestly and courageously uses his intelligence and fulfils the duty to express the results of his thoughts in clear form."*

What do you see when you look upon a naked person? Do you see a penis, testicles, breasts, or vulva or do you see a person, a real living breathing individual who has genuine emotions and wants to be accepted, loved and cherished like everyone else? Does the sight of reproductive parts define that person, does the fact of visibility change anything about that person? Am I a penis on legs or am I a human being? Reports in the gutter press about naturists often concentrate on "the wobbly bits" or use language that concentrates on body parts. Naturists concentrate on people.

History

Why did we ever invent clothes?

The earliest evidence of the use of clothes is somewhat controversial but maybe stems from about 20,000 years ago in the stone age and consists of figurines carved from stone and depicting a garment of unknown type. The function of this garment appears to be associated with fertility rather than modesty. The first practical use of clothes was for carrying items. [7] Men wore a belt to help carry objects, leaving arms and hands available for hunting or defence. As hunter gatherers, they would have travelled large distances so carrying would be easier with hands free and they would be better able to protect themselves. Whilst the men hunted, the women gathered food and tended the children so early clothing for them consisted of aids to hold berries etc. They may also have carried their babies in slings. This is not only an ancient practice, in recent times the Andamanese people were photographed wearing just such items of apparel. Having become more adept at using available materials, men would have used clothes for protection of their genitals, these being prone to injury whilst hunting. It was only as climates changed that the need for clothing to provide warmth and protection would have become more important. As peoples migrated to inhabit other areas, they encountered colder winters where survival depended not just on a good food supply but on the ability to keep warm. In warmer places, this did not occur so the manufacture of clothing was driven by the desire for decoration and the display of social status. The use of clothing did not arise from a sense of modesty, that only came later with specific middle eastern religious beliefs.

All this is still much in evidence today but the tribes that live in the warmer parts of the world vary a good deal regarding clothing. The Yanomami tribe in Brazil spend much of their time nude with the exception of a string-like belt worn by the men into which their foreskin is clamped. The females of the Nuer people in the Southern Sudan wear bands around their waist to show the wealth of their father. Their breasts and genital area are open to the air. When they wish to act in an erotic way, then don leather skirts! The nearby Dinka people are similar, the idea of visual modesty taught in the west simply has no meaning there. A TV program made by Jeremy Bradshaw in the 1990s for the Survival Specials [9] series showed the current plight the Dinka people. Their way of life is being changed by a new canal under construction across their tribal lands. The programme showed the Dinka people engaged in all sorts of activity from social gatherings to herding their much prized cattle. Much of the time they were naked but both men and women occasionally wore some clothing. There did not seem to be a consistent theme for when they did or didn't wear clothing. The point is, nudity was not an issue. Other tribes such as the South American Quechua do use clothes, but the idea of nudity in public is not the same as it is in the West. Those who swim in the river or go about other quite normal activities can do so nude without any censure, they may wear clothes at times for specific purposes but in contrast with the West, being seen nude is not an issue. To them the idea of a naturist club would be incomprehensible, clothes are for fun, ceremonies, tribal status and art.

Clothes have been used as status symbols for a very long time. High status individuals would mark their position by wearing specific items of clothing. In the reign of Edward III, the huge fine of 40 shillings was imposed on anyone if they wore shoes exceeding a certain size yet were not a Lord, esquire or gentleman. This was to maintain the strength of the status symbol and more importantly, the power and influence of the wearers.

The association of nudity and modesty only came about as a result of the religious teachings of early Jewish and Christian sects, many centuries after the introduction of clothing for practical purposes. They taught that sex was a sin unless it was without enjoyment and only for procreation. Nudity was seen as directly related to sex so was included in their strictures. Once clothing had become commonplace and the very restrictive religious rules were in place, people became very adept at providing sexual signals by other means, often using clothing itself.

Famously, King Henry VIII used large codpiece to highlight his genitals that in turn underlined his masculinity and power. At various times over the years, female breasts have been displayed either uplifted and shown with an obvious décolletage or squashed and hidden in the manner of the 1920s. Legs are either hidden behind flowing skirts or displayed to the hip as at the height of the mini-skirt fashion in the 1960s. Even modern strip clubs and purveyors of porn use clad women, not nude, the clothes used and the manner in which they are worn suggest sexuality of all kinds. People who live naked use sexual come-on signals to attract a mate but nudity of itself is not sexually stimulating. This can easily be demonstrated by a visit to a naturist establishment, there you will not see large numbers of folk in a state of sexual excitement. That is not to say that naturists don't have sex, of course they do, the point is that simple nudity is not sexual.

The coming of the habit of clothing at all times has not stopped sexual signals as the religious teachers would have liked, it has simply made people adopt new and often cunning means to signal sexual desire whilst remaining dressed. They can be used for modesty but can also be used to make statements about the individual, either for status or sexual purposes. Far from providing simple modesty, clothes provide a huge range of sexual come-ons from the subtle to the blatant. This is recognised in extreme religious sects such as the Taliban, this sect require that every part of the woman is hidden to prevent men from being driven sex mad. Even the eyes must be hidden as it is well known they can be used as a sexual come-on. Their teachings are quite old, they come from the same Jewish and Christian teachers that taught that women were a source of evil and that sex was an abomination. All fun leads to sin.

Every part of the body has been taboo or not at one time or another. In some cultures, the feet are thought to be more erotic than breasts so are more carefully hidden or displayed depending on intention. In others, the neck is thought to be highly erotic so is hidden to all except lovers. The penis of men in New Guinea is highly accentuated with a large curved sheath, the larger ones belonging to the higher status males rather than those who have the larger penis.

Clothing and its use as a status symbol is not only the domain of important people. Modern business suits are a direct descendant of clothing used purely as status symbols. Their origin lies in the hunting jacket. People who did not need to work because they were sufficiently well off to support themselves, had time and money enough to hunt. Others who did work took to wearing hunting jackets as an indication of assumed or implied status. This became widespread, such jackets are now part of the ubiquitous business suit. Apart from the very modern introduction of Casual Friday, business suits are assumed to be vital, those who break the code are likely to be shunned in favour of those who conform. The signal it gives is *"I'm safe, I am one of your tribe"*.

As Desmond Morris points out, some aspects of human behaviour have lasted a very long time without any conscious effort. [10] People are creatures of habit, they do it because they were shown that way, not because it is rational or sensible. This replicated behaviour is now described in terms of memes and is the subject of a later chapter. The wearing of clothes is one such behaviour, we cover up determinedly out of habit even if the temperature makes this very uncomfortable. Another example of how ideas and habits carry on through the centuries without any particular reason they should do so is the famous rude two finger sign. This is made with palm inwards and two fingers thrust upward, it originated in 1415. When English archers fought the French at Agincourt, they were under threat of having their index and middle fingers cut off by the enemy, should they lose the battle. These fingers were used to draw the feared longbow; showing that the two fingers were still there was an act of defiance. This gesture is in common use still today, although most will have no idea of its origin.

There is no biological basis to feeling one must cover up at all times, the behaviour is learned and goes in a cycle, being constantly reinforced. It started in the distant past, a few Jewish and Christian religious zealots taught that sex and therefore nudity was sinful unless it was for procreation only, women were classed either as second class humans or as temptresses. The zealots taught that conforming to their rules would lead to infinite pleasure after death. Many people reacted by obeying these teachings as the majority of a population are followers not leaders, a fact that people like Hitler and Stalin used to their advantage. It is a sad reflection on life that so many follow and do not think for themselves, if they did, most of the odd and dangerous regimes around the world would never have come to power. Once the Catholic Church was established, force was used to make many conform, fear did the rest. With this regime in place, the almost sex (and therefore nude) free life was transmitted to children who grew up and did the same to their children. The threat of punishment on earth and for eternity was sufficient for the idea to be taught again and again. Anyone who may have felt like a nude swim would not have done so for fear of sin, punishment or ridicule. The desire to be free from this depressing cycle was not strong enough to overcome these teachings until the Western decline in religious fervour, a strong factor in the start of social nudity in Germany. Even without a prominent religion, people will often not change, even if change is an excellent idea. There are many who live by habit, they keep the old ways because that is "how it is done". They teach that to their children and the cycle continues.

In "Mark Twain in Eruption", its famous and much quoted author wrote *"We are discreet sheep; we wait to see how the drove is going, and then go with the drove. We have two opinions: one private, which we are afraid to express; and another one - the one we use - which we force ourselves to wear to please Mrs. Grundy, until habit makes us comfortable in it, and the custom of defending it presently makes us love it, adore it, and forget how pitifully we came by it. Look at it in politics."*

The point is clear, there is no fundamental reason to enforce modesty with clothing. The reason such behaviour is normal in the western world is due solely to the reinforced habit of dressing carried over from parent to child over the centuries. It has become a meme complex of amazing strength. As Desmond Morris says: *"Despite the many fascinating variations that exist from region to region and society to society, every one of the thousands of millions of human beings alive today shares an almost identical genetic inheritance. We may wear different hats but we all show the same smile; we may speak different languages but they are all rooted in the same basic grammar; we may have different marriage customs but we all fall in love. Despite our different skin colours, religious beliefs and social rituals, we are biologically astonishingly close to one another."* [9]

With the decline in the repressive authority of the Catholic Church, the Western World is changing but the cycle is being broken only very slowly. Any changes in society take a long time unless there are huge forces such as the Great War 1914-1918. Here, various social values changed permanently. Out went the direct unquestioning submission to authority, in came a new awareness of politics for the common man. Women had to wait a while longer for universal suffrage but change was in the air. The 2nd World War brought even more changes. Since the start of the naturist movement about 100 years ago, there are now millions of people who enjoy at least some aspects of a socially nude lifestyle, all that is required now is the legislative bodies and the police to catch up with the change in society. This will be easier in Europe, the USA has a very great deal of catching up as the Christian Right are very vociferous and often hold positions of considerable power. Their record is not impressive. Issues such as racial segregation, the unilateral imposition of power on helpless countries and the huge number of poor in the USA are all testament to their failure, as is the very high rate of sexual deviancy, teenage pregnancy, gun crime and murder.

Naturists have broken this habit by being rational. They have recognised that questioning the whole reason for clothes has not provided a convincing case to keep them under all circumstances. There is a role for clothes, for protection, fashion, status, fun and in some instances, modesty, but there is also a place for nudity. Some very keen naturist campaigners would argue for universal nudity but they will never achieve this. In my view, the ideal would be a world where books such as this are not required, where nudity is simply not an issue. I am not saying that nudity should be the norm in the high street, the supermarket or the bank, I am saying that in appropriate places and times, nude people should attract no particular attention.

A brief history of modern naturism

In the modern western world, organised social nudity started in Germany, then a new nation built from a coalition of city states. It had only recently been at war with its neighbour France, resulting in a social climate far from settled as far as the population was concerned. In hindsight, the roots of the both the first and second world wars were already in place. Empire building leaders such as Bismarck sought to make Germany the leading nation in Europe.

The roots of social nudity came from right and left wing politics in Germany at the very end of the 19th Century as part of the Lebensreform or life reform movement. In the 1890's a German youth league called Die Wandervogel (migratory bird) was started in Berlin. Its members promoted the ideas of fitness and vigour and looked back to Teutonic ideals of nationalism. Although Germany had been the victors the Franco-Prussian war in 1870, the humiliation of French victories over nascent German states prior to that encouraged a military outlook and the nation was ready for huge social upheavals that would only end in 1945 after both World Wars. The youth that joined the Wandervogel wanted to throw off the restrictive views of their elders and to rediscover nature from which they felt they had been alienated. It was common to hike in the woods, bathe in the lakes or simply to bask in the beauty of the countryside, but more importantly, to cast off the old social ways. It was just such an idea that encouraged them to swim and walk naked, this was at least partly as a protest at the old restrictions. The movement was huge but lack of a national organisation makes it difficult to gauge just how huge it was. They never formed an effective political force because one aim was to forget the effects of their parent's politics, hiking and swimming were more important than lobbying.

At more or less the same time, some doctors of the Naturheilbewegung, (Natural Healing Movement), were treating diseases such as TB, rheumatism and scrofula with exposure to sunshine. To be effective, the patients would be nude. This treatment, heliotherapy, would later be used to treat soldiers injured in the Great War.

At the start of the 20th Century, an artistic movement called Die Brücke, (The Bridge) started. A key member was Germany's most prominent exponent of German Expressionism, Ernst Ludwig Kirchner. Die Brücke consisted of artists searching for an honest response to the zeitgeist (spirit of the time). Kirchner wrote in his diary *"It was lucky that our group was composed of genuinely talented people, whose characters and gifts, even in the context of human relations, left them with no other choice but the profession of artist...The way this aspect of our everyday surroundings developed, from the first painted ceiling in the first Dresden studio to the total harmony of rooms in each of our studios in Berlin, was an uninterrupted logical progression, which went hand in hand with our artistic developments in paintings, print and sculpture... and the first thing for the artists was free drawing from the free human body in the freedom of nature."* [11] His studio was a free and liberal place to be, the nude models were not professionals but came from the artist's circle of friends, nudity was celebrated. Artists in Die Brücke frequented the Moritzburg lakes near Dresden. Here nude bathing was became very common, they would paint landscapes and nudes in an atmosphere of free expression.

In 1912, Kirchner wrote *"(they) stripped of their clothes and civilised trappings, the artists and their models were at one with nature and led the lives of modern primitives."* Sadly Kirchner split from the movement and then suffered a severe physical and psychological breakdown in the Great War. He killed himself for his art after being declared 'degenerate' by the Nazis in 1937.

In this climate of change and renewal, one person who promoted such ideas and those of improved social hygiene was Heinrich Pudor. Just before the turn of the century, this Doctor of Philosophy published a books such as Nackende Menschen, Naked People and Jauchzen der Zukunft, Naked Mankind, both of which became very influential. These were followed by The Cult of the Nude considered by some to be a classic work. Apart from promoting nudity as a treatment for a range of ills, it also outlined the mental and emotional benefits of naturism, as long of course that participants followed the rather austere life it described. A little later, the politically right wing Richard Ungewitter published a book along similar lines, it was entitled simply Die Nacktheit, Nakedness. From its publication in 1905, this book sold over 90,000 copies; no doubt the sales were improved by the illustrations it contained. He followed this with the start-up of a nudist society called Tefal, an acronym for Treubund Fur Aufsteigendes Leben, the Confidential Lodge for the Friends of Rising Light. Tefal promoted the ideas in his book, a Utopian view where everyone would be naked, eat only vegetables and abstain from alcohol and tobacco.

Anyone putting such ideas forward now might be associated with the New Age but other aspects of his philosophy had a darker side. Members had to be Germanic, blue eyed, blonde. Aryans. It is easy to look with post holocaust hindsight to see the evil contained in this aspect of Pudor's ideas. Although the Nazis did not promote naturism, some tolerated it. Others did not but they did promote the idea of a Aryan race and committed the most evil acts in history to achieve their goals.

As has been said many times, history is like a foreign country, they do things differently there. At the same time that right wing nudist culture was becoming widespread, the left wing used social nudity to further their ends. Adolf Koch, a left wing primary school teacher, sought to use social nudity in a new political movement to free people from *"authority-fixated conditioning which held proletarians in deference to their masters: parental authority, the paternalism of school and church, the mass media, and the organs of law and order."* [15] He used "organic-rhythmical exercises" in his Berlin schools in the early 1920s. The conservative press formed a campaign against him but, with the support of the Prussian Social-Democratic government, he was able to build up schools dedicated to his methods, eventually having some 3,000 pupils. The nudists went on to become a huge element in the left wing politics of Germany. A subsection of the huge Worker Sports Organisation was the Proletarische Freikoerperkulturbewegung, the Proletarian Naturist Movement and numbered at least 60,000 members, a larger number than those in the right wing naturist associations.

Another interesting character of the time was Werner Zimmermann from Switzerland. He preached against body guilt and encouraged naked education. It is easy to see a darker side now in the light of the current paedophile scare; one can imagine the headlines if works such as his were written and published in this climate, after all, he favoured nudity at school! To do that would be to entirely miss the point, Zimmermann's philosophy was to eliminate body guilt, encourage openness and end what he saw as the cause of sexual deviations such as paedophilia. In his view, it was repression of the human spirit that was the root of sexual and relationship problems. Honest nakedness ends curiosity about bodies and encourages a healthier attitude to sex and bodily functions.

At this time of social change the world's first nudist resort was opened. It was started by another Zimmermann, although not related to Werner. Paul's project was named Freilichtpark or Free Light Park and was sited in Lubeck, north east of Hamburg. It attracted people from all over the world. It was open only to those serious in their beliefs in Nacktkultur, naked culture, and was run on a strict basis.

All this work stopped with the outbreak of the Great War in 1914. At the end of the war, Germany signed an Armistice, but this proved to be a surrender. The terms of the Treaty of Versailles made it worse and humiliated Germany and opened the way for Hitler and his evil ideas. In the 1920's the Wandervogel continued, at least partly as a release from the crushing poverty, unemployment and humiliating conditions under which many lived in Germany. If one was poor, nude swimming in the lakes was free as was nude hiking, the fellowship of like-minded people helped to shut out the horrors of everyday life.

Both left and right wing political activists used social nudity in the inter war years to further their own separate aims. Nacktkultur thrived, not just in Germany, centres opened across Europe, New Zealand, Australia and even in that most prudish of countries, the USA. In 1929 a Congress of Nudity and Education was organised by Adolf Koch.. He had been acquitted by a court for teaching nude gymnastics but the case made him famous and it was this fame that helped to attract over 3000 people to the Congress from all over the world. It was widely reported in favourable terms in most newspapers. Times had changed. A contemporary of Koch, one Major Hans Surén was teaching his soldiers to do their gymnastics nude. After five years the Army sacked him, but this only provided the time and impetus for him to write Mensch und die Sonne, Man and Sunlight. It sold in huge numbers and had to be reprinted 61 times in just 14 months from February 1924.

Times changed again, this time for the worse. The 2nd World War put an end to Nacktkultur, at least in the directly organised way that started before the Great War. After Goering banned all non-Nazi organisations, Himmler, once again allowed the practice of nude sunbathing, but such was the situation in Germany that nothing significant developed until after the 2nd World War when naturism or Freikörperkultur (FKK, Free Body Culture) took off again. With another period of unemployment and poverty, nudity is a free way to enjoy life and it is seen as a means to purify the soul and rid oneself of war guilt. There are a large number of clubs but more importantly there are parts of public parks where nude sunbathing is commonplace. The attitude in modern Germany towards public nudity is a very healthy one, the local authorities now promote the lifestyle and it has lost its political connotations. Indeed some concern has been shown recently by the local authority in Hamburg at the diminished number of nude people using the parks. This is a result of increased tolerance of nudity, people do not feel they have to go to a special place anymore to be nude and enjoy the sun and air.

Oddly, in the country where naturism started, some local authorities are attempting to restrict nude bathing on the more popular beaches. Before re-unification, East Germans enjoyed social nudity as a cheap way to enjoy themselves in a poor economy. Now the country is reunified, popular Baltic beaches such as Warnemunde have become packed with West German tourists, some of whom dislike nude culture. In an attempt to reassert their former influence, Catholic and Protestant activists are persuading local tourist officials to restrict nude recreation. Changes in attitudes are never uniform and those that reach the media are often driven by those keen to get the publicity. German remains a nation more at ease with nudity than most others.

The UK

The ideas that spread from Germany became known as Freikörperkultur, FKK or Free Body Culture. In England, there had been a tradition of nude bathing in the less populated areas, often just men and poor men at that, but sometimes mixed. Victor Hugo and his mistress Juliette Drouet were surprised to find mixed nude bathing in Guernsey when they visited in 1873. Widespread organised nudity did not come to England until the 1920's when the ideas being developed in Germany caught on. A man by the name of H. D. Byngham start the English Gymnosophist Society, gymnosophist and the modern word gymnasium being derived from the Greek word gymnos meaning naked. Following the loss of their facility at Wickford in Essex, they changed their name to the New Gymnosophist Society and produced England's first naturist magazine. An early member of the society was N. F. Barford who along with others, helped acquire 4 acres of ground at Bricket Wood in Hertfordshire. It is still in use by naturists today.

For much of the 1920's the naturist movement grew in England, even attracting positive comment in the newspapers. One or two attacks by outsiders such as Nesta Webster resulted in those in the movement becoming more secretive; it did not stop them following their beliefs, they simply withdrew into the woods. It also resulted in their using pseudonyms to protect member's true identities. Translated versions of the German publications, books from English and foreign authors all helped to further the cause. One by an anonymous American even had the temerity to mention the role of sex in naturism, he wrote *"As a matter of fact, gymnosophic association is much more satisfactory than in clothed society, because both sexes can see everything they crave and no disturbing feelings are aroused by irritating and unwholesome concealment".* He was brave to link these two subjects at a time when some would act in a violent manner simply when some men sunbathed in public in just shorts. This violence occurred at one of the most celebrated events in English naturism.

It happened at the Welsh Harp in what is now North London. The Welsh Harp comprises land and a lake, some of the land was privately owned at the time. Members of the Sun Ray Health Club and New Life Society indulged in semi-clad and nude sunbathing in the hot summer of 1930, led by an ex-Army Captain, Harold Hubert Vincent. Following a silly season article in a newspaper, angry protesters turned up to harangue them, even though they were on private property and well away from any public area or footpath. The police were called on a number of occasions and had to protect the naturists as they were not breaking any law and were vulnerable to the violence from the crowd. The publicity from the so called Sun Bathing War resulted in widespread sympathy for the naturists, far from removing them from the area, the protestors actually helped them. They should have known, the English nearly always side with the underdog and they hate injustice.

When land near the Bricket Wood camp came up for sale, another key individual in the English movement took his chance and bought it. Charles Macaskie sold his business to raise the funds, he and his wife Dorothy moved onto the land with a tent and precious little else apart from a few tools and the conviction to make it work. They called it Spielplatz or Play Place. In 2004 it is still a centre for owner occupiers to life a permanently naked lifestyle.

Naturist clubs in England open all over the place, they kept themselves to themselves, organising first as the Central Council for British Naturism then simply as British Naturism. They have followed the secretive, "ping-pong in the woods" style of naturism and hence have failed to attract a wider audience, especially younger members. Naturism in England is changing, attitudes are improving as more and more discover the pleasures of social nudity when at foreign holiday destinations. There are thought to be more than two million people in England who have made this discovery, most would not describe themselves as naturists as they have no desire to be linked with the traditional clubs, none the less, they are more accepting of nudity and hence are happy to swim and sunbathe nude in the company of friends and families with the benefits that brings.

France

It was the French who coined the name naturism or naturisme as they would spell it. This was in 1778! In the 1920s, it really took off in France, it remains one of the best naturist destinations in the world. The La Fédération Française de Naturisme, created in 1950, now brings together 160 associations and 85 holiday centres. For a strongly Catholic country, France welcomes naturism. French Government Tourist Office actively promotes naturism at the many centres around the country.

Croatia and the Former Yugoslavia

Following the 2nd World War, the countries that made up the former Yugoslavia had every reason to hate the Germans and it is greatly to their credit that German naturists have been welcomed in large numbers.

The official story of organised naturism in Croatia starts in August 1936 on the island of Rab. King Edward VIII stayed on Rab and was allowed to take nude swims in the bay of Kandarola accompanied by his wife, now the bay is sometimes called the Engleska Plaza (English Beach). The island had been used for nude bathing long before that, at the turn of the 19th Century Rab was used by naturists and there was accommodation for 50 or more. Croatia was the first country in Europe to have commercial naturist resorts. Koversada opened its gates for nude leisure in 1961, adding to the 100,000 total places for those who enjoyed nude holidays in Croatia. Naturism is strongly supported by Croatian government bodies but most naturists in Croatia are not Croats, it is estimated they number less than 5% of all guests in naturist resorts. Compared with the situation in 1980's, the number of organised naturist resorts in Croatia has decreased owing to the effects of the Catholic Church. The Croats who do try to live a nude lifestyle prefer unofficial or secluded beaches.

The USA

In the same year that the Welsh Harp wars were in full swing, the American League for Physical Culture was born. Taking their ideals and example from Germany, people such as Bernarr Macfadden and Kurt Barthel started organised nudity in the USA. As in other countries, the authorities took a dim view. In one incident, a small group of Barthel's ALPC friends were practising gymnastics at a gym in New York. The police broke down the door and arrested the people inside. When it went to court, the magistrate threw out the case, they were doing nothing wrong.

As is usual with controversial court cases, the publicity surrounding the incident resulted in increased interest, organised nudity increased. By 1933 there were centres in 5 states and by 1936 there were over 80 such centres. It was different on a public beach. In a hot summer in the 1930s, a thousands of men had the temerity to go topless on Long Island NY, all breaking the law. It is hard to imagine now a society that banned topless bathing by men.

A rival to the ALPC was started by a disgruntled member. Uncle Danny, whose real name was the Rev. Ilsley Boone, started The International Nudist Conference. Just as well for a country late in the field of naturism, they dropped the International part of their title as they did not speak for other countries, the INC became the American Sunbathing Association. Uncle Danny's influence and power grew until he felt he was in an unassailable position. Having waited for the horrors of the 2nd World War to pass into history, dissatisfied ASA members ousted Uncle Danny was a coup. He stared another organisation but it never prospered, the ASA went on to represent most nudist clubs in the USA, a position it still holds. Unlike the Spartan life espoused by the Germans, the US clubs went for comfort. Many are run as profitable commercial concerns. The ASA is now called the American Association for Nude Recreation, AANR.

Sadly, the USA is also home of ultra-conservative Christians, many in positions of power and influence. These people see evil in practically any strand of life and one of their favourite targets are nudists. For a country that claims to be the home of freedom, it is hard to understand just how repressive the culture has remained since the puritanical Pilgrim Fathers. Outsiders know the USA far from being the land of the free but it is interesting to compare their experience with that of Europe. In France where nudity on public beaches is hardly an issue, their rate of sex related and violent crime is a small fraction of that in the USA. A trip around a video shop showing US titles will give great cause for concern, the majority have at least some violence, most show no nudity at all. As Christianity has peace and goodwill to all as a core belief; how can a country that preaches these values produce such an imbalance and at the same time, persecute naturists who try to lead a peaceful life? How can the same country also revel in violence in its culture and its foreign policy and still claim to be a freedom loving Christian country? There is a clear difference between claim and fact.

In the modern USA, prudery reigns [12] Females are generally not allowed to show nipples even whilst breastfeeding although New York State have legalised exposure of women's nipples on grounds of equal protection to men. There is the related campaign for of "topfree equality" that is being pursued on constitutional grounds of equality of the sexes. It seems likely that suppressed sexuality is one of the root causes of the strange prudery seen in the USA. A visit to any video hire shop will at the very least make you suspicious, most of the titles on the shelves will celebrate violence and the projection of US power by violent means. All these are at the eye level of children. Any "adult" titles in the shop will be kept away from children. Nudity is seen as more harmful than bombing women and children. The oddest thing about this attitude is the placing of titles that deal with naturism. Although there are not many naturist videos, they will be with the adult titles just as magazine sellers keep naturist magazines on the top shelf alongside the porn.

In US made films, the Hayes Code that was used from the 1930s until the 1960s defined what was and what was not allowed to be shown. Since 1st November 1968, this has given way to the MPAA film rating system but full frontal nudity is still rare. This is in contrast to the prevalence of violence, some of which is extreme. The MPAA system allows children to see films that many would consider too violent but not those depicting nudity. US TV is more prudish still. Nude scenes in theatrical films are edited out or obscured in some fashion. There is nudity in some films but it is almost always related to sex rather than to naturism. There is also nudity in art in the US but many works have been removed or covered in a similar manner to the 19th Century Victorians in England.

Australia

There have been several reports in the past of when the aboriginal people in Tasmania were given clothes by missionaries, the gifts were accepted graciously. As they did not share the body shame of the religious Westerners, they took delight in undressing at moments calculated to embarrass the priests. Cases of kidnapping occurred where the captured European was examined to see what they were hiding, the aboriginals being puzzled by the discovery that there was nothing different. [13]

Modern Australia shares many of its attitudes to nudity with the UK. In Western Australia the naturists living in Perth won a notable victory. A stretch of beach between the sea and the Special Air Services base was used by nude people for recreation. The local authority took action in the courts to stop them. When the court ruled that it was the Army who had jurisdiction, the authority tried to get the Army to stop nude activities. As it had no effect on the efficient running of the Army, the soldiers took no action. Now the beach, called Swanbourne, is the scene of much nude activity, quite outside the reach of the local council. It seems this is like the UK where a few vociferous folk in a position of power have not listened to their electorate. Huge numbers of people use the beach, the people have voted with their feet and there has not been an large local uprising against the nudes. The council had not listened nor made the effort to become more in line with the wishes of the public.

In Queensland, a hot area ideal for nude living, the State Government has banned public nudity and the police enforce this. In a land famed for its love of an outdoor life, this seems odd, especially when considering of the large amount of money that could be made from providing naturist facilities.

Japan

Until western influences caused a change, it was common to see communal nude bathing in Japan, it still happens where people wish to retain a very traditional way of life. Japanese magazines were not allowed to show nude photographs but that situation has changed, at least a little. The An An magazine asked its readers to send in nude pictures of themselves, the 1600 women who responded saw the photographs as complimentary not salacious. This idea is interesting, nudity is not the issue, the assumption is not made that nude images are automatically pornographic. It has been the west, mainly the USA, that has given rise to the idea that nudity is always sexual, always sinful and must therefore be repressed.

The dark side of naturism

Sex crimes

There is a website by Nikki Craft [14] headed "Exposing Nudism & Naturism's Dirty Little Secrets". This site lists some disturbing items, mainly concerning paedophiles and their arrest. Assuming the information is accurate, Nikki Craft is helping to highlight a key point about naturism, i.e. when sexual deviants like paedophiles go to naturist establishments etc., they are easier to catch than when in the rest of society. Deviant behaviour is far easier to spot in a nude environment and thankfully it is far less common than in communities that promote repression.

As has been seen in the recent past, some priests of the Catholic Church, mainly in the USA, have been found guilty of gross indecency and paedophilia. The repression of sexuality is a large factor in the cause of this deviant behaviour, and the teaching of body shame is a direct cause of the secrecy by the victims, they felt they could not speak out and seek help when attacked by those thought to be in a position of authority. It is interesting to note that Nikki Craft does not attack naturism itself, the idea of wholesome nudity, she attacks deviant behaviour, behaviour that is considered deviant anywhere in society and naturists would agree with her.

She says *"Early in my involvement in the upper echelons of the naturist movement it became apparent I was running into a large number of paedophiles, child molesters, child pornographers and their apologists; disturbingly disproportionate for such a small, fringe group. I had never run into such a consortium of men, in various ways, abusing children; and never have since, either."* It is clear the she joined the naturist movement and was sufficiently committed to join the upper echelons. It was only after running into a large number of sick people that she left, presumably to take up the forever dressed life again.

This seems to be a problem in the USA, a country known for its promotion of violence and repression of sexuality. Nowhere else has this been reported as a problem specific to naturist organisations. On the contrary, anyone even thought to be odd is removed. She does go on to outline her opposition to all aspects of sexual crime and sexual exploitation of women. Good luck to her in that respect, that is an uphill struggle. The exploitation of women has its root in the same ancient religious teachings that sex is bad, women are temptresses etc. Sadly she fails to see the positive role that naturism plays in this. The promotion of body acceptance, of openness about nudity and of life in general all work in direct opposition to such things. Who would pay for nude photographs if nudity was commonplace? Secretiveness promotes pornography, sin sells it.

Fascism

The early days of Nacktkultur in Germany are badly coloured by unfortunate political views. Although the left wing element, followers of Adolf Koch and others, were a large proportion of the nudist movement, there was a significant number of nudists who believed in the developing ideas of National Socialism. The political and social climate of the time can be seen in hindsight to have been the fore-runner of Nazi "theory", not just the Holocaust, but all the other dreadful acts they perpetrated. The dark side of Nacktkultur was the insistence by Ungewitter and others on Aryan members of the movement, the blue eyed blondes much favoured by Hitler and his compatriots.

Even though Ungewitter and his apostles favoured an Aryan membership, in 1933 Hermann Goering banned all organised nudity in Germany. He wrote *"the naked culture is one of the largest dangers for the German culture and morality. It is expected therefore by all police authorities that they seize all measures in support of the mental forces developed by the national movement, in order to exterminate the so-called naked culture. The naked federations of culture must be supervised. In so far as institutes of bath or grounds were placed at the disposal, it is necessary to influence on the owners that the contracts are solved."* [15]

Goering did not think Nacktkultur fitted in with the perversions of the Nazis and Hitler said "Nudity is undignified and an error of taste" but in the Nazi party, there were many sympathisers towards nacktkultur. They saw it as a means of promoting the

Aryan ideal, so following the closures by Goering, the leader of the SS, Heinrich Himmler, gave the instruction to the Gestapo in 1936 not to obstruct the practice of nude sunbathing any longer. [16] Two areas in Berlin were released again officially for naked bathing and the Freilichtpark near Lubeck survived. Of the two arms of the nudist movement, one survived. The ultra-right wing element died with the end of the 2nd World War, the remaining left wing element survived but has mutated into the essentially non-political FKK movement in modern Germany.

Society at large

What naturism means to different people

It is best at the outset to say what naturism is not. It is not pornographic, it does not support paedophiles or any other sexual deviancy and it is not about swinging. Very sadly, deviants have used the words nudist or naturist to describe their wares, especially on the internet. An internet search for "nudist" will yield the address of real nudist websites but it will also lead to all sorts of material that has nothing to do with what is described in this book, the simple enjoyment of a naked lifestyle. Neither is it about show, people exhibiting themselves, to see and be seen; it is not about display. People use dress for that, donning the right clothes to suit rank, status, class or tribal allegiance.

The words naturist or nudist conjure up different notions in different people. This private meaning of the word is part of what has become part of each person's idiolect. An idiolect is similar in some respects to a dialect, it is the set of more personal meanings, images or ideas associated with words. To some, a naturist is someone who lives a normal life but goes away at weekends to a "nudist colony" and "prances around naked". The activity is secretive so breeds rumours of odd practices; the more secretive, the wilder the rumours.

The mass media often fuel this nonsense, with ludicrous double-entendres. They will print things like *"You can't hang out there"* or *"We'd love to see more of you"* or even *"Bottoms up"*. They do not really know what happens, and use school boy humour to describe pubescent ideas. The Carry-On films made this worse. One in particular, Carry On Camping, depicted two men who decide to spend a camping holiday at a nudist camping site with their less than enthusiastic girlfriends. The venture is a failure but not until all the old prejudices have been wheeled out. No doubt it was thought to be funny at the time but now it is simply boring. Newspapers in the UK have recently printed items more sympathetic to naturism, they have even sent reporters to take part, some of whom have been converted to the way of life, others have seen the sense even if they choose not to join in. The television companies have also improved, driven no doubt by the increasing size of the naturist movement and their realisation that there is good business to be had.

To others, a naturist is a mysterious person who feels the need to go back to nature. They are likely to be vegetarian, they would not smoke or drink alcohol but would lead lives without many of the comforts of modern life. This approach started in Germany at the beginning of the 20th century as part of the German Lebensreform or life reform movement . Books by left wing activists like Heinrich Pudor and right wingers such as Heinrich Ungewitter pursued these ideas. These publications presented a Utopian view of life in total nudity. When the Nazis banned all non-Nazi organisations, nudism in Germany withdrew into illegality but flourished again after the war ended in 1945. The ideas behind naturism became more popular but as the numbers grew, people started to want more comfort and to leave behind the Spartan camps. Holiday centres opened that did not require membership and the old naturist clubs shrank. Some of these old clubs are still running but with much reduced membership because they fail to attract sufficient new blood. So as the older members leave or die off, they are not replaced, but their ideas die with them. In a new trend, some of these clubs are now being purchased and run as commercial concerns. Gone are the committees, rules and hide-bound attitudes of the old guard, these are being replaced by brighter modern facilities aimed at attracting everyone.

The modern idea is that a naturist is simply someone who has lost the need to wear clothes at all times. Far more naturists now belong to this group than the old naturist clubs. People can take a holiday at large nude resorts such as le Cap d'Agde in the south of France where up to 35,000 nude people can enjoy a regular holiday supported by shops, restaurants, banks, supermarkets, pools, bars, marina etc. all without clothes. The numbers of people in Europe that spend at least part of the life nude now runs into many millions. The USA is a long way behind, they are still wrestling with the social memes set in place by the Puritans, but even there, things are changing.

Some people feel quite strongly about not being part of a naturist club. As Shane Steinkamp says, *"I don't see the point in going to a club where the only thing I have in common with people is that I don't have any body shame. Of course, if the club goers actually didn't have any body shame, then they probably wouldn't be hiding in their little clubs anyway, so the whole existence of the nudist clubs seems to me rather like an opium den."* [17]

Memes and Naturism

Modes of social behaviour are governed by memes, i.e. learned ideas and attitudes. A meme is described as *"An element of a culture that may be considered to be passed on by non-genetic means, esp. imitation"* [18] Richard Dawkins first came up with the idea of memes in his book "The Selfish Gene", 1976. [19]

Dr. Susan Blackmore puts it like this: *"This means that whatever is copied from person to person is a meme. Everything you have learned by copying it from someone else is a meme; every word in your language, every catch-phrase or saying. Every story you have ever heard, and every song you know, is a meme. The fact that you drive on the left (or perhaps the right), that you drink lager, think sun-dried tomatoes are passé, and wear jeans and a T-shirt to work are memes. The style of your house and your bicycle, the design of the roads in your city and the colour of the buses - all these are memes."* [20]

There are good memes, those that benefit the holder or others and there are bad memes, those that cause a bad effect on one or more people, sometimes including the person holding the meme itself. An example of a good set of memes is found in nurses, doctors etc. the idea that helping the sick or injured is imperative, they simply would not walk by on the other side of the road at the scene of an accident. This is a learned response, people that care for others often come from families and friends where such care is the norm. The *"always care"* meme is transferred by deliberate teaching or by example but can also be transferred by unconscious means. The important point is that the idea itself replicates. Had the same person been brought up in a criminal environment where brutality and violence were the norm, an injured person would not pose a threat so walking on by would be thought normal, even sensible. Criminal behaviour transferred from parent to child in a seemingly endless cycle has been a serious social problem for centuries, the memes that drive this cycle are bad but very successful. It has long been argued that good is more powerful than bad, that in the long term good will triumph over evil. If this is so, it will depend not on any heavenly intervention, it will depend on the relative success of good and bad sets of memes.

Memes are not simply thoughts, a thought such as *"I am hungry"* or *"that is a lovely flower"* is not a thought that replicates, it is not a meme.

Once identified as bad, a meme can have its success reduced but rational means, but the really successful memes are very difficult to eliminate. Some people will still tell you that getting your feet wet will *"give you a chill"*, i.e. give you the common cold. It has been known for years the common cold is caused by a virus and not by cooling the feet with water but the meme survives, despite rational effort, it replicates from person to person.

A successful meme lives on in society for a long time, possibly centuries. They replicate by various methods; they may mutate but still live on. A successful meme does not imply that it is good or bad, it is simply able to replicate and survive in a manner similar in behaviour to a physical virus. The virus that causes the common cold is very successful, efforts to rid the human race of this irritating organism have failed. As a virus it is very successful even though most people would rate it is as bad! Another example of a successful meme is belief in a God. Note this does not imply how good a meme is, merely success. A very bad set of successful memes was strongly promoted by the Nazis and rational teaching

41

has largely eliminated these bad memes but some are still successful, sadly one can find individuals around the world busy infecting others with them. Another bad but successful meme is *"smoking is cool"*. It replicates well but kills off its carriers. It replicates by a number of methods, not generally by being taught, it is more subtle that that. Millions are spent by tobacco companies on these subtle methods to ensure the meme stays alive.

A related set of memes is known as a meme complex, groups of memes mutually supporting each other and replicating together. The lifecycle of a meme or meme complex can be compared with that of a virus. A person that carries a meme, the vector, infects a new carrier. The new carrier either accepts the meme or rejects it, they are either susceptible or immune. The original vector can now die, if the new carrier was not immune, the meme lives.

Clearly naturism is a meme complex, it is learned behaviour. Naturists would argue this behaviour provides significant benefit and is therefore good but its success as a meme complex is less clear. Although millions have now tried and liked at least some aspect of a naturist lifestyle, counter memes are very strong in their effect. The counter meme is that which causes people always to be dressed, even under extreme circumstances, reinforced by religious memes that cause a feeling of guilt about bodies, enjoyment or sensual experience.

Why is the dressed meme complex more powerful than the naturist meme? Because it is reinforced from childhood and fuelled by inappropriate sanctions. Consider the behaviour of adults when supervising children. If some 2 year olds are playing in a private garden, the adults would consider it quite normal for the children to play nude, even if people outside of the immediate family are present. If other children are brought along, they will happily join in nude and no-one would think a problem existed. As the children get older, both boys and girls will be encouraged to wear some kind of covering but the children will often abandon them as useless. As they get older still, parents will become more insistent, telling the children it is required to wear something, the children eventually accept that as the norm, they will also have seen that their parents are never nude in the garden even if they may see them nude at bath time. By now the children have learned there is something of a problem about parts of their body, an idea that would not have occurred to them had they not been taught. The meme is being reinforced all the time. In this situation dressing is not for warmth, comfort or status, it is for something beyond the understanding of such youngsters, but as they are generally accustomed to obeying their parents, they comply. By now it feels normal to wear clothes when playing in the paddling pool or in the garden. Unless these children are brought up in a naturist environment, the *"always dressed outside"* meme will rarely be in competition with an *"its ok to be nude"* meme. The dressed meme is by then firmly established.

Parents will feel that even though they have no objection to children playing nude in a private back garden, they will wonder what the neighbours will say, what friends may think if they visit such a household. Fear will play a part, fear very much increased in the present panic over paedophiles. Paedophiles are dangerous individuals, children must be protected from their perverted behaviour, but this protection must not be at the expense of the children themselves. Sadly this is just what happens, the always dressed meme is reinforced in all manner of ways by parents, neighbours, friends, TV etc. As they grow up, being always dressed will seem normal. The always dressed meme is supported by the "others will think us funny" meme if any nude activities go on in places visible by outsiders.

This has developed into a very successful meme complex, one that self-replicates with amazing robustness. Even though when asked, many adults will say they have no argument against nudity from an intellectual point of view, they would not participate for emotional reasons, their memes are more powerful than rationality. To reinforce this and to make their memes even more successful, those who say *"I don't mind if other people are naked"* will almost invariably say *"but I realise that most other people will object"*. This dual nature of their meme complex is perhaps the central reason it is so successful at replicating. When naturists challenge this view, the results are surprising. In England, about nine tenths of those asked thought naturists were harmless [21] but the second part of the meme will still cause very effective replication, *"stay dressed not for me but for others"*.

Since the start of the naturist movement, the idea of social nudity has increased, even in the face of very successful counter memes. There are two reasons for this, first that from a rational point of view, naturism is enjoyable and harmless so people work out for themselves that nudity is fine, secondly, those individuals who have discovered the benefits of naturism have actively promoted the idea. Such promotion is another means of meme replication.

Susan Blackmore again: *"Some memes succeed in getting copied because they are good, useful, true, or beautiful, while others succeed even though they are false or useless. From the meme's point of view all this is irrelevant. If a meme can survive and get replicated it will. Generally we humans do try to select true ideas over false ones, and good over bad; after all our biology has set us up to do just that, but we do it imperfectly, and we leave all kinds of opportunities for other memes to get copied - using us as their copying machinery."* [19]

It is this idea that humans try to select the good over the bad that has resulted in a rise on popularity of a naturist lifestyle. In competition with other successful memes, a rational selection process is slowly increasing the success of the *"its ok to be nude"* meme.

In terms of memes, it is interesting to look at cults, if only because one of the very first publications on social nudity was Pudor's "Cult of Nudity". In this sense, a cult is a meme-complex characterised by self-isolation of the infected group, leader-worship, brainwashing by repetitive exposure and genetic functions being discouraged, e.g. celibacy. Naturists certainly isolate themselves but more for the sensitivity of others, not because they wish to be isolated. In what might be called modern naturism, there is no trace of the other four factors that describe a cult in memetic terms. There is no convincing evidence to suggest that all very early naturists were cult members, but in any case, the movement has changed considerably since then.

Some people, searching for their identity after a traumatic discovery have been heard to express the sentiment that *"In order to understand my future, I must understand my past"*. In terms of memes, what they are saying is that they have missed out on assimilating the memes of their past. If they do not feel part of the social group they feel they "should" belong to it is because they have yet to gather all the memes of the group. Going back to a mother country or culture helps to absorb such memes and hence to reduce the contrast between themselves and that culture, they feel more at home.

Attitudes in Society

What is outside yourself does not convey much worth; Clothes do not make the man, the saddle not the horse. Angelius Silesius [22]

The attitude found in society at large to social nudity varies a good deal from country to country and from time to time. After journeying from Monte Video in the mid-19th Century, Charles Darwin witnessed a Gaucho control a restive horse in the water. He wrote *"A naked man on a naked horse is a fine spectacle; I had no idea how well the two animals suited each other."* [23] Following a visit to the Argentinean port of Bahia Blanca he wrote *"The old Indian father and his son escaped, and were free. What a fine picture one can form in one's mind, -- the naked, bronze-like figure of the old man with his little boy, riding like a Mazeppa on the white horse, thus leaving far behind him the host of his pursuers!"* [24] The prudery common in the Victorian era was not spread equally across society, any more than the much touted freedom we are supposed to live under is evenly spread in modern society.

Fashion, image and spin

A bigger problem than prudery for the naturist is the trend towards presentation over content, what looks good is good regardless of other evidence.

A visit to a magazine shop or the viewing of an average evening of TV should be enough to convince anyone that fashion, image and spin are hugely popular. Whilst much of this is quite harmless, the darker side cannot be ignored. Anorexia and bulimia are serious illnesses and are very common, they are brought on or made much worse by the relentless quest for the perfect body. The models used to show the latest fashions are thought to be almost perfect, little do people realise the pain these people go through to achieve this, nor do they realise the efforts that go on in magazine production offices to make them look flawless.

Modern computerised photo retouching can have an amazing effect. Photographs in the glossies do look flawless, but they are made to convey a message, not to portray a person. What you see is an attempt by the very skilled to make you believe in an image. It is a modern form of what went on in churches in decades past, believe and you will find happiness, do not believe and you will become an outcast.

Many people actually suffer as a result of this, they will not take part in all sorts of activities because they feel their body will not fit in. Typical victims are those who consider themselves to be overweight being unable to go swimming, simply because their body image does not match the fashionable one. This is a very sad state of affairs, humans being devalued by a fashion culture. To make it worse, those who feel the need to hide behind their carefully designed image will feel the need to ridicule the more relaxed and self-confident nude people in order to justify their own pre-occupation with image. There is a degree of smugness in their behaviour, they think they are "in" so feel able to laugh at outsiders.

What people really think

In January 2001, a survey by NOP Solutions on behalf of British Naturism reported only 1% of people would call the police if confronted with public nudity. 88% of people interviewed thought naturism was "harmless". It seems from this evidence that most people are happy with nudity, the problems for naturists come from a vociferous minority, some of whom assume they are the modern thinkers and that most others would be offended by nudity. They are not likely to be swayed by evidence, their beliefs are what drive them on. A more complete summary of the NOP poll is shown in the Appendix but one question was *"Naturists enjoy activities such as sunbathing and swimming without clothes. Do you think such people are: criminal, disgusting, harmless or sensible?"* The result was: harmless 88%, sensible 40%, criminal 2% , disgusting 7%. This is a very interesting result and quite in line with discussions I have had with people from all over the world. Sadly it does not seem to be in line with the attitude taken by law makers and the police, but they are not known for being in tune with the public that pays their wages.

In Britain, a number of naturist clubs have started to hire their local authority's swimming pool for naturist swimming sessions. Some authorities would not comply, using all the old prejudices as good reasons why they acted as they did. Those who did comply were surprised at the popularity of these events and that nothing immoral or odd was taking place. In recent years, some other local authorities, seeing the success of these events, have now approached their local naturist clubs to run such events. What a turn round!

A similar change in attitude has occurred with regard to local nude beaches. In 1979, part of Brighton beach on the South coast of England was designated as a nude beach. This was a brave step for the local authority and they weathered some vociferous protests from a few people. Despite this, the beach celebrated its 25th anniversary in 2004 and naturists still have the backing of the authority. Money speaks, the authority have realised the popularity of naturism and the money it brings in.

In England there is an active group of naturist walkers. They plan routes in the countryside well away from buildings and people and surprisingly are able to walk nude for miles in the open air. They do not seek to be a campaigning group and they dress if someone is encountered enroute. Considerable effort is put into planning the walks so that others are not offended. In 10 or 12 years of running these walks, no problems have been encountered. It is inevitable that others are encountered occasionally but most do not realise what has happened, they see a group of people walk by, the group has seen them first and covered up. Sometimes this is not possible, the person is not seen in time and there follows an encounter with 10-40 people with nothing on. Some smile and bid good afternoon, some seem bemused but do nothing, one or two watch as the nude walkers recede into the distance. There are some of course that would like to join in.

On one occasion, a farmer on a quad bike saw the group emerge from the edge of a wood and could not believe his eyes, a mixed group of nude people in the sunshine. He drove off but came back to make sure he was not dreaming. By this time the group had covered up and were happy to talk to him. He had not heard or even dreamed of such a pastime but was clearly tempted to join in. Far from being outraged, many are envious of the freedom of thought and action of those who walk naked.

One of the group members who has more experience than most of nude walking has described many encounters over the years, none of them troublesome. Following one encounter, a family out for a picnic even invited him to join in with them, asking questions about naturism and congratulating him for his courtesy. This is a huge difference from what the vocal anti-nudity protestors may have predicted for this type of encounter. They would have drawn dark pictures of crime, unusual sexual practices etc. and of course the "damage" to the children, even though they would be unable to produce any evidence to support their claims.

Is Nudity in adverts always acceptable to naturists? Not at all. There is nothing wrong with nude people of all shapes and sizes but often nudity is exploited to achieve a sensational effect or even to continue the selling the idea of the perfect body. I would like to live in a world where nudity is not an issue, adverts that use nudity to cause a sensation simply reinforce the fact that it is an issue so to me are not acceptable.

Nudity is fine, exploitation is not. There has been a recent set of complaints from naturists about nude calendars. These show nude firemen or cricketers but their genitals are always hidden in what is intended to be a humorous manner. Whilst mainly harmless, these photographs highlight the "naughty parts" whilst keeping them hidden, reinforcing their supposed naughtiness.

Prudery from Victorian times to the present

The story of how the Victorians modestly covered the legs of their pianos is a myth. [25] Thomas Pyles' book Words and Ways of American English contains what is claimed to be the most likely explanation, that an English traveller by the name of Captain Frederick Marryat invented the story as a joke. He wrote it in his book, Diary in America. It is a wonderful story if you want to exaggerate the idea of Victorian prudery, especially US prudery. The problem with reports of prudery or any other single behaviour type, is that it is unlikely to be uniformly spread across the whole country and across a whole time span, human society is more complex than that. The prudery of the Victorian age predates Queen Victoria herself, she reigned 1837 until her death in 1901. A visit to her home, Osborne House on the Isle of Wight, will be a surprise to anyone sure of her prudery, the house contains a wonderful collection of nude statues and works of art. You could be excused if you thought that far from being prudish, Queen Victoria had a very accepting attitude to nudity.

Research into sexual attitudes in the Victorian era does not show agreement on the general state of prudery, rather such research shows there was no universal set of attitudes held by "the

Victorians". There are cases of extreme prudery to contrast with cases of openly lewd and lascivious behaviour, there are the moral crusaders and the campaigners for a more broadminded society. In a world without effective contraception and with a deal of ignorance about pregnancy in general, abstinence from sex makes sense, especially with the often crippling economic burden of too many children. It would be easy to slip into the *"sex is sin"* frame of mind, sex brings problems so sex must be bad even if this attitude is not supportable by plain common sense. It is not the case that the Victorians were universally prudish, it is that some of the more forceful people promoted prudish attitudes for a variety of motives. Public nude bathing was common on the beaches of the UK by the 1840's.

A more likely explanation of Victorian prudery, one that has more power if you remember that it predated the Queen, is that establishment prudery came about as a side effect of running the Empire. French colonialists made a habit of taking a local bride, indeed it was encouraged, English men in the same position often took a local mistress, especially in India. These mistresses were not accepted in English society in India but they were often celebrated in art. The English establishment saw this as a threat to their power. It was feared these foreign women would weaken the influence of the ruling white men, so fraternisation became frowned upon.

As it was sex that drove these men to take a foreign mistress, sex itself was seen as be bad, it had to be stamped out. This continued past the end of Victoria's rule, as an example [26], in December 1908 a Mr Scoresby Routledge M.A. wrote a letter to the Times newspaper reporting that a British official in Kenya, an Acting District Commissioner, had two native mistresses. As a result of this letter, the press reacted strongly, a typical reaction being an editorial in the Spectator of 12th December where the editor wrote: *"The empire will be ruined if officials use their powers to gratify their animal passions. The accepted standard in East Africa is lower than in the empire as a whole and has reached a point of peril"*. The uproar resulted in a Circular Directive to all overseas British officials, it was written by the Colonial Secretary of the time, Lord Crewe, warning officers *"that such practices were damaging and unworthy and led to scandal and grave discredit"*.

The Spectator editorial recorded that the "mistresses" were just 13 years old, one said to be "unwilling", the other being removed to be under the protection of a "native" policeman. In modern terms, the British official was a paedophile, but at the time the uproar was about damage to the Empire, not the poor little girl. If the empire had been safe, the fate of the girls would not have been recorded. The Government in the form of Lord Crewe, Routledge and the newspapers were not primarily driven by prudery, all worried more about the empire and the maintenance of British rule than the people involved.

It cannot be a coincidence that during the puritanical Victorian age, there was a huge sex trade, especially in London. In 1859, the Lancet reported that there were 2,828 brothels in London and probably 80,000 prostitutes. Some or even many of these prostitutes were children, they were poor, disease ridden and starving. Repression simply makes some people secretive, they react against repression, sex and every aspect of the body becomes devalued, a meat transaction rather than a demonstration of any kind of love or affection. I conclude from this that repression is always harmful and leads to more not less immoral behaviour.

Prudery can be funny. During a visit to America, Winston Churchill attended a buffet luncheon at which cold chicken was served. Returning for a second helping, he asked politely, *"May I have some breast?"*

"Mr. Churchill," replied the hostess, *"in this country we ask for white meat or dark meat."* at which Churchill apologised profusely. The following morning, the lady received a magnificent orchid from her guest of honour. The accompanying card read: *"I would be most obliged if you would pin this on your white meat"*

As an extreme example of the prudery in the USA, there is the Janet Jackson incident. At the Super Bowl halftime show on 1st February 2004, her right breast was briefly seen on TV. The US public and press went to town and gave an excellent demonstration of their dreadful prudery. Jackson had an invitation to perform at the 2004 Grammy Awards cancelled and a lawsuit was filed by one Terri Carlin *"on behalf of all American citizens who watched the outrageous conduct.".*

The lawsuit was dropped but the incident also triggered other legal action. This action resulted in fines for companies involved with the broadcast. Even the law was changed, the Federal Communications Commission is now able to fine up to $500,000 per violation instead of the original maximum of $27,500. Europeans reported this and took the opportunity to laugh at America's expense. A typical report said *"How reassuring to the rest of the world that the U.S. has its priorities straight. We, the poorly informed old Europeans, wouldn't have realised that Jackson's breast was a more important issue than Iraq's missing weapons of mass destruction. But the U.S. media is covering the breast-baring incident like the story of the century."* Frankfurter Allgemeine Zeitung.

Children

Soon the child's clear eye is clouded over by ideas and opinions, preconceptions and abstractions. Simple free being becomes encrusted with the burdensome armour of the ego. Not until years later does an instinct come that a vital sense of mystery has been withdrawn. The sun glints through the pines, and the heart is pierced in a moment of beauty and strange pain, like a memory of paradise. After that day, we become seekers. Peter Matthiessen [27]

It is especially interesting to witness the effects of naturism on children. They take to it without reserve. As they grow older, the habit of hiding behind clothes is taught by others. Any parent will know how often their children will cast off their clothes in the summer without a thought. Naturism helps children become well balanced adults with healthy attitudes to their bodies and to others. Unhappily, the current scares about paedophiles are causing much anguish. It is now much harder to bring up children as well balanced people with healthy attitudes. The unhappy beings who prey on children should of course be locked up, but a bigger problem is how to protect all children from their corrosive effects, not just their direct victims.

In a very real sense, all children have already become their victims, all of them are being damaged by some of the very silly attitudes that are becoming more common. Teachers cannot put their arm around a distressed child, they must be left in their misery to avoid the accusations of frightened parents. Children cannot be led by the hand across the road for the same reason so are at a greater risk of being mown down by traffic. The rule in some schools is that children are never to be touched in any way. It is even suggested that parents have a permit to photograph children at school events.

This is utter madness and will backfire on the very children that people are seeking to protect. Naturism offers respect for people's bodies, respect for the people themselves. I suspect strongly that paedophiles had a restricted, perverted upbringing and their disorder has been made much worse by repression. I fear greatly the impact of the current madness, I fear we are breeding more and worse paedophiles. The prudery on the Victorian age did not prevent the huge number of child prostitutes. Openness about humans and their bodies must be better than repression and secrecy.

If this madness gets worse, parents will be banned or at least feel inhibited to have their young children in the bath with them as has been the practice over many decades. Even without embracing a naturist lifestyle, children from families where nudity is the norm, at least in certain circumstances, will be better able to make meaningful relationships, form loving, open sexual partnerships and be more contented human beings.

Babies are not only born naked, they are born happy about their bodies. It does not worry them if they are naked, the very concept does not exist in their mind. In the process of becoming an adult, an individual must learn that their nude body must be hidden away except in certain highly contrived circumstances. It may seem odd to describe having a shower as a highly contrived circumstance, but consider the shower room where it takes place. There are locks on the doors to prevent unauthorised entry and obscured glass at the window to prevent anyone seeing. The placing of the room in a house is away from the main thoroughfare for the same reason, to keep nude people out of sight. There is a difference between the need for some privacy and spending considerable sums constructing sight proof rooms where nudity is allowed.

As Dorothy Rowe points out in her book Successful Self [28], not everyone can be trusted when it comes to telling children how to behave. She was told by her mother that when entering hospital, *"the sooner she stopped crying, the sooner you'll go home"*. She stopped crying immediately but did not go home soon afterwards. Children told that covering up is necessary are only told a half truth, it is more important for the parent that the child is covered, not for the uncomprehending child. To these parents, covering up means more than modesty, it means hiding oneself away behind a façade.

Some parents will fear adverse reactions from others especially now in the general panic over paedophiles. The *"quick, get dressed before the neighbours see you"* will reinforce the body shame in children but this does not have to be the case. When my children were quite young, they played nude quite happily in the garden. On one occasion friends came with their two girls, both of whom where some years older, perhaps 10 or 12. The eldest girl was well into puberty but was keen to join the little ones in the pool, it being a hot day. It was pressure from the smaller children to undress and get in the pool, the visiting girl did not have her swimming togs so not going nude meant missing out on the fun. Although she was a little shy at first, all played nude quite happily. Just because bodies change, a child is still a child for a long time. Their parents were a little surprised but happy to let them continue. No harm was done, rather, I would argue the experience was good for all, it helped to build a positive body image.

In 2001 the Saatchi gallery put on an exhibition that consisted of photographs taken by Tierney Gearon of her children and in just two of the images, the kids were nude.

The newspaper "News of the World" attacked Gearon and set off a police investigation under the 1978 Protection of Children Act which in turn led to a court case. This Act, which makes it a criminal offence to take an indecent photograph of a child, is aimed at protecting children from abuse. The case failed as it was clear that no abuse had taken place, any perversity being in the eye of the beholder. Apart from the News of the World stunt to sell more papers, it is disturbing to note the attitude of the police and prosecuting service, the CPS. They seem to view all pictures of naked children as being perverted in some way, that everyone that takes such photographs must have had a sexual motive. In this case, many well-known people came to the support of Gearon, even Chris Smith, the then Culture Secretary, a senior member of the Government. It seems odd that the police and CPS can be so out of touch with what most people think. During a TV programme called Taboo, Gearon said to the presenter, Joan Bakewell, *"You know what's fascinating is I received quite a few letters from parents that had children that were abused by paedophiles and every single one of them said 'do not let them take those pictures down'. What are we going to do, are we going to cage our children up, you know, are we going to put them in cages and hide them inside, in our houses and not let them out?"*

Breastfeeding and childbirth

Naturists are happy with nudity and do not share the "hide at all costs" attitude common in Western society, but they generally understand why non-naturists cover up. What is beyond understanding is why anyone should think that a mother breastfeeding her child should be considered unacceptable. Even in cultures that choose clothing for much of the time, breastfeeding in public is common, normal and is a very beautiful sight.

In 2004, a law was passed in Scotland to prevent anyone interfering with a parent feeding a child, the Act specifically mentions mothers breastfeeding. Now anyone who tries to make a breastfeeding mother move on or stop feeding will face a large fine. It is a shame that a law is required to achieve this end but at least the legislative body had the common sense to do so. With luck the sight of women feeding their babies will soften the hearts to those daft enough to oppose the bill. In a TV programme reporting on the Scottish legislation, a man in a restaurant was heard to say *"who would want to see a women feeding a child while I have my dinner"*. This astonishing opinion was held by someone forgetting that the baby was having her dinner! He had the mistaken idea that breasts are wholly sexual in nature, he did not realise that breasts are sexualised because they are usually covered, they are not covered because they are sexualised.

Serious consequences of body shame

Doctors in the UK and the USA have reported cases of people with advanced symptoms of diseases such as colon cancer. These people are hard to treat and often die as a result of their late presentation. Prudery, body shame and sheer embarrassment have prevented them from reporting the early signs to a doctor, ensuring that the possibility of early and therefore successful treatment is reduced. They will have effectively "died of shame".

Terrorist counter measures may require nudity in the process of the cleansing of noxious substances. Some people would rather die from the effects of chemicals than be exposed naked to the gaze of strangers. The emergency services have to make separate facilities for male and female victims of gas attacks, increasing their workload for no net benefit. In a society where nudity was no real issue, such ideas would not arise making the sad but necessary work much easier.

Circular Arguments and Paedophiles

In 1918, the Asian 'flu killed millions of people. As scientists then had less understanding than today about how 'flu is spread, people reacted by spraying all sorts of chemicals over almost everything. Sadly it did little good, people still died. Faced with such an emergency, there was a desperate search for a solution and many hit out in all directions, all to no avail. Much the same is happening with the paedophile scare. Although it is clear these perverts must be kept away from children, it is quite wrong to panic and hit out at any aspect of human behaviour that may be rumoured to be connected. Circular arguments are used to justify such panic, they go like this, "Dogs like chocolate. You like chocolate, therefore you are a dog". The usual daft argument put forward about naturism and children is "Paedophiles like nudity, you like nudity, therefore you are a Paedophile".

In his book "I am Right, You are Wrong". Edward DeBono gives two very nice examples of circular arguments, the first goes like this: *"A very talented journalist friend of mine will walk twenty floors up to a New York party because she has a phobia about lifts. She is not afraid of the lift breaking and rushing to the ground but of being trapped. Whenever she looks at a lift she sees only a place in which to be trapped. The chances of being so trapped are probably less than choking on a piece of steak, but perception does not compute statistics."* [29] His second example is: *"One farmer (nationality omitted) said to another: 'You see the trails made by those planes high up in the sky. Well, they are trying to make rain. I can prove it. You never see them on cloudy days, do you?'"* [28]

Of the first story, he makes the point *"if you always avoid the situation you fear, you can never get enough experience of it to show that your fears are groundless."* This applies most cogently to those who have never even contemplated being in a socially nude environment, if you don't know what it is like, how do you know you would not enjoy it?

"Give me the child until he is seven and I will show you the man". Often attributed to Ignatius of Loyola [30], this famous quotation indicates how pliable children are. When taught before the age of seven, the core Memes are laid down. In a Catholic family these Memes would include *"you belong to the one true faith"*, in an American family it would include *"You live in the best country in the world"* and in too many families, *"you must cover that part of your body at all times"*. Paedophiles use this aspect of a child to groom them into behaving in a way desired by the pervert. They rely on secrecy and carrying on their perversion on private. In contrast, naturism promotes the idea of openness, body acceptance and a healthy attitude to sex, an approach to life directly opposite to the secret perversion of paedophiles. As mentioned before, nude sexually excited men are easy to spot, it is the always dressed world that has suffered the highest incidence of paedophile damage to children.

Beliefs and Religion

In the ancient world, public nudity was common, or at the very least, it was not thought of as being significant. Attitudes to sex and nudity were very different from the modern Western view. As far as naturism is concerned, I use this to illustrate the point that there is no inbuilt human characteristic that works against public nudity, it is simply learnt behaviour. Humans are all the same regarding their biology, the innate way they work, what differs between cultures is what is learnt as people go through life, what attitudes they are taught and what is considered to be right and wrong. To understand other societies or times gone by, it is important to set aside preconceptions of our own society and to look at the art and writings in a detached way.

As Leslie Poles Hartley said, *"The past is a foreign country; they do things differently there"* [31] Yes they do, but they were all human, all the same under the skin.

Attempts to control language or to enforce a given definition on words will always end in failure. Whilst I might make a distinction between the words erotica and pornography, it does not mean that others will agree or even understand without explanation. I would use the word erotica to mean sexually arousing in a worthwhile and enjoyable fashion whereas pornography is everything that devalues sex, making it a commercial transaction without regard to love, warmth or human emotion. I fully realise that many use both these words interchangeably. Sadly there is nothing I can do about that.

Every human culture has a means of explaining life and why we are here. Amongst other things, each explanation will tell how and why we were created. Many cultures explain creation in sexual terms, fertility and sexual union being seen as wholesome. Westerners who look upon the art of such cultures tend to interpret sexual scenes in a Western sense, as erotica or pornography, they fail to see the meaning as it was intended. The depiction of an erect penis would shock many, especially those from the USA where such an image leads to anxiety and embarrassment, but to many cultures, the erect penis means fertility and hence life. It has even been used as a good luck charm. An example of this is a Romano-British pot from the 2nd or 3rd Century CE found in Cambridgeshire which has a phallic decoration. [32] It was believed to promote good luck and avert evil.

What follows are a few examples of when and how such attitudes were different. In the British Museum can be seen an Egyptian painting on papyrus from circa 950 BCE [33], showing what to western eyes is the nude figure of sky-goddess Nut after having had sex with the god Geb. In fact, the scene symbolises resurrection as well as Nut's part in a basic creation myth. The image is appropriate to the burial chamber where it was found. Also in the British Museum is the Warren Cup [34], a Roman silver wine-cup from the 1st century BCE or later. It shows a man with a nude male youngster. In the beliefs held at the time it was made, the homoerotic scene conveyed power and status as well as simple desire. This cup would not have been hidden away like some pornographic object. Guests to the house of the owner would have seen it as being normal, just like some of the wall paintings at Pompeii that depict sexual scenes. The final example from the British Museum is part of a relief from a 10th Century CE. It came from a Northern Indian temple and shows an amorous couple. [35] The imagery shows the human soul seeking union with the divine, not a pornographic object of desire. To the modern western eyes, what is clear is the lack of shame or guilt, the lovers are truly lovers engaged in an act of spiritual power.

In ancient Egypt during the reign of Pharaoh Akhen-Aton (1385-1353 BCE), athletes competed nude, people exercised and studied whilst nude. Dr. deHoratev said of Akhen-Aton and his queen Nefertiti " ..that not only the Pharaoh and his wife but also their children and officials went around with too few clothes (transparent at that!) or no clothes at all, that they practised nudity in the royal palace, in the royal gardens and swimming pool, that they loved physical beauty, valued good food and wine, and led a frankly joyful existence." [36]

From ancient times in Japan, bathing was used for religious purposes, to cure injuries and for enjoyment. In the Shinto religion, they used the term Kamiyu (Divine bath) for the hot mineral springs by the sick and for purification. In the Edo era (1603-1867) Sento public bathhouses were popular. Sento was part of a sophisticated culture, a place used to meet one's friends, neighbours and strangers as well as a place to get clean. The baths were mixed gender and it was not the Japanese way to care much about body image, at least not in the modern Western sense; a body was a body. As a result, the Japanese term Hadaka no tsukiai came about, it means "the best friends are the friends of nudity" or "naked companionship" or "naked acquaintances", usually in the sense of best friends. The widely practised nude communal bathing continued until recently, even now some mixed public baths still exist in small villages in the deep countryside.

Five Christian groups from the 2nd to the 15th century practised public nudity: the Adamites, Adamianis, Carpocrations,

Encratites, and Marcosians. Ascetics in ancient India such as the Diganbara sect of Jainism also practised nudity as part of their quest for simplicity.

Anti-nudity

Religious teachings are at the root of anti-nudity ideas. They are also the source of the related anti female teachings, the consequence of which has been the long term subjugation of women, a struggle in which proponents of universal suffrage and feminism are still engaged.

Religion has much to its credit but also much to be ashamed of. On the credit side, religious believers have often managed to bring a more peaceful life to parts of the world when decline and violent struggle were very common. Many find that religious ideas bring order and understanding to a turbulent world. In contrast, most religions, supported by their hierarchies, have used underhanded political means and brutal violence to achieve their aims and consequently have themselves added greatly to the turbulence of the world. A visit to art galleries in Bruges in war torn Flanders makes the point quite well, the depiction of religiously inspired torture and death is prized, innocent nudity is missing.

Religion is always controversial. It is not my intention to put a case for or against religion or for a God, merely to put the case that the larger religions do not have anything even approaching a coherent view on nudity.

One problem one must face when considering religious attitudes to naturism is that there are no universally agreed views on nudity, even within what appears to be one religion. In a more general sense, a brief study will show a key feature of organised religious life, disagreement. It seems it is just not possible for a single large group of people to hold collectively one set of beliefs. The history of religion is characterised by schism, once a group of believers grows above a certain size, it will split into two or more groups and each new group will claim they are guardians of the fundamental truth. As each group grows, each will schism into more and more sub groups. A current example is the Church of England. For what some would like to be taken as a "whole" religion, the Church of England is in fact a loose collection of groups of people who may share some beliefs but who also harbour fundamental differences. Attempts are made to keep the depth of these differences out of the public eye but recent battles over women priests and homosexuality have thrown them into sharp relief.

Members of the church need not be alarmed, this is the normal state of religious organisations, a permanent state of flux. Some would even argue this is the proper state in which to be, a state that converges on ultimate truth, but this imagined convergence has been going on for centuries and there is still no end in sight. This endless cycle of schism has produced a huge variety of sects in all the religions of the world and there have been many more in history, some dying out after only a brief existence, others lasting centuries. Hardly a day goes by when a report is not shown in the media of some religiously inspired act of violence, one lot trying to gain ascendancy over others.

That is not to say religion causes all conflict, far from it. Hitler and Stalin were two of the most evil people who have ever walked the face of the earth. Both caused war, misery and destruction but not as a result of religious beliefs. To achieve any understanding of history, or at least how power was obtained and maintained, one must acknowledge the effect of religious belief on conflict. Far too often conflict is caused purely by differences in such beliefs. By conflict I do not only mean shooting wars, I include the hate that splits communities, causes misery, poverty and death by starvation and disease.

Extreme examples are to be found in Northern Ireland where even within "one side" of the Catholic/Protestant divide there exists a whole range of opinion from peace loving to murderous or in the Taliban of Afghanistan whose treatment of women is impossible for Westerns to tolerate. All these differences result in a very wide variation of religious attitudes to nudity but as Aldous Huxley wrote, *"The propagandist's purpose is to make one set of people forget that certain other sets of people are human."*

How can religion sway the behaviour of so many? We like to think we live our own lives following our own free will, but many don't. Too many people follow others, they do what they are told. Many will accept the guidance of religious teachers almost as fact on the grounds that the teachers have studied religion for years, therefore they know better. This attitude is very odd in a society where freewill is said to be valued, instead of a person joining a religion because they agree with its principles, they agree with its principles because they are a member of the religion! In the case of naturism, they may have enjoyed a nude swim with their family whilst on holiday in Europe, but on return to their own country, have encountered opposition to social nudity from their church.

They are told what to think so act accordingly, they never do it again. The problem lies in handing over the business of sorting out what is right and wrong to religious teachers, some of whom have ideas that run directly against common sense and human biology. As there is no universal set of teachings even inside one religion not matter how hard the leaders work to achieve it, relying on a few teachers to define what is right and wrong is dangerous, everyone should decide for themselves. In " A History of God, Karen Armstrong makes the point nicely, *"…many of the people who attend religious services in our own society are not interested in theology, want nothing too exotic and dislike the idea of change.... They do not expect brilliant ideas from the sermon and are disturbed by changes in the liturgy".* [36]

Those that believe but do not think about their beliefs, will hand them on to their children. These children may reject the direct outward signs of belief such as church attendance, but will retain some of the habits like never been seen nude except in very specific circumstances, so the old Christian teachings go on and on without thought. Whilst many accept religious teaching without question, this is not universal. As an ex nun, Karen

Armstrong said, *"The more I learned about the history of religion, the more my earlier misgivings were justified. The doctrines that I had accepted without question as a child were indeed man-made, constructed over a long period of time. Science seemed to have disposed of the Creator God and biblical scholars had proved that Jesus had never claimed to be divine."* [37] She had discovered that what was taught as fact in school was simply the collected beliefs of a few.

This is directly in line with my experience in Catholic schools, we were told that the Catholic faith had lasted 2000 years because it was right and that it had stood up to rigorous questioning. What the teachers missed, many of them nuns, was the fact that during much of those 2000 years, no-one was allowed to question it! The other point they missed was the fact that the Church they represented and whose doctrines they taught was very different from that of 2000 years earlier.

Far from lasting 2000 years, it had changed, split and re-organised many times. It had undergone periods when stoning to death was thought to be the right thing, periods when killing non-Christians was to be rewarded in heaven and periods when tiny children were told they would rot and burn in hell if they told a lie.

The irony of the last point was lost on the nuns. Once a religion is established, by whatever means, its memes are strongly set in the minds of the community. They will be transferred to the children who become the new carriers, later to transfer them to their children in an endless cycle, a cycle reinforced by churches, schools etc. Once such memes are in the people's minds, they breed automatically. Much the same can be said about other human activities, for example, the famous Senegalese conservationist Baba Dioum is often quoted as saying *"For in the end we will conserve only what we love. We will love only what we understand. We will understand only what we are taught."* [38] He was talking about conservation but the same principle applies, people believe what they are taught to believe. It takes an effort of will to change.

The other way that religions have extended and maintained their influence, both in the past and in the current era, is the direct use of violence. Even now in many parts of the world, if an individual runs contrary to the prevalent religion they risk being ridiculed, ostracised, imprisoned, tortured or killed. The more extreme religions use the most extreme means. It is little wonder that people obey the rules. Leaders will then claim they represent the majority and that what they teach is therefore "right". Eventually these regimes fall as they always have in the past not without conflict and misery. If you doubt these assertions, just watch the news.

I do not wish to be anti-religious because there is plenty of evidence to show that religions can and do have a beneficial effect on society and on individuals, indeed this is one strong reason they prosper. Most Western religions agree on the core ideas, one God, peace and good will to all, care for the sick etc. Even the Eastern religions are not different in every respect, some may believe in several Gods but peace and care of the sick are still core to their teachings. The outward signs of a religion have been laid on top of core beliefs by centuries of change.

For example, nowhere in the bible or other religious books does it describe in detail the lavish ceremonies that take place with priests dressed in very expensive clothes in opulent cathedrals. As Thomas Fuller said, *"Many come to bring their clothes to church rather than themselves."* [39] On the contrary, most espouse the idea of humility as a core belief, but the way that organised religion has developed has hidden these beliefs under layers of widely differing practices.

All religions offer a set of beliefs, values and philosophies. Atheism does not make these offers, those who call themselves atheist simply do not believe in a God but there are plenty of people who do not believe in God and who would not describe themselves as atheists, they shun the idea of an "ism". It is an oddity of language that non-belief in a God is called Atheism. As there is no coherent set of beliefs, it cannot be an ism, rather it is the lack of belief that is the main characteristic. For this reason there is no atheist attitude to nudity, atheists are a diverse group of people.

I find it odd that some atheists still cling to religiously inspired attitudes especially those regarding nudity and the place of women in society. Whilst being able to present a strong argument about the non-existence of God, many are at a loss to know why bodies are seen as shameful and why women are still often treated as second class citizens. It may come as a shock to find that ancient religious beliefs are the source of both these attitudes and they are supporting them by spreading the memes.

A central claim made to support atheism is that religion stops people thinking in a rational and objective way and forces them to rely on outside authority, rather than becoming self-reliant. As there is no rational argument to insist on clothes at all times, it would seem obvious that atheists would be naturists, but the two ideas only come together in a haphazard manner.

As far as this book is concerned, the differences of interest are those concerned with nudity. The differences range from an extreme Islamic view that all women should be covered, even their eyes, to the Diganbara sect of Jainism where nudity was the way of life. The current Western Christian position also shows very wide differences, from the ultra-prudish Christians in the USA, some of whom have been campaigning to dress nude statues, to the Christian naturist associations that preach that Christ was crucified nude and that nude living celebrates His life.

What has all this to do with naturism?

1. If you believe in a God, can you in all humility say that His creation is so seriously flawed that it must be kept hidden? Did He get it so wrong that each and every one of us must hide at every point in case someone else, equally flawed, might just see us? Of course one cannot look to organised religion to answer this question as you will get widely differing answers, you must decide for yourself.

2. Have you knowingly or otherwise taught your children they should be ashamed of their bodies. If so, did you question these teachings or have you simply accepted them? If so, why?

3. If you do not believe in a God, does the power of religious belief in maintaining the always dressed meme have any relevance to your life? Are you happy to accept the result of other people's religion without question?

4. If you believe that always being dressed is "the norm", would you consider the norm to change over time? Most realise the "norm" does change but few think about the means by which it changes. If you are convinced by the intellectual case for nudity, what would your reaction be to seeing a nude person at your local swimming bath or working in their garden? These are the people who are the engine of change, are they wrong?

The Romans and the Christians:

The Roman view of religion was very different from the modern Western Christian view. They had many Gods but each was not of the same character as the Christian God. When Christianity started as a Jewish sect, it was accepted in Roman society just as any other sect, indeed a key feature of Roman occupation was tolerance of previous or differing religions. The Christians taught their beliefs but these were also very different from those heard in churches today. A key difference relevant to the subject of this book is that women were valued and not seen as temptresses bent on the destruction of men, a view taken by Christians only centuries after the time of Christ. Christianity grew only very slowly into a separate gentile religion but all along, it has changed.

Bathing in ancient Rome was a communal activity for people of all classes, conducted in public baths similar to modern spas or health clubs. Apart from just bathing, going to the baths was a good excuse to indulge in gossip or to do some business. There was also an intellectual side, some of the baths (thermae) had libraries and lecture halls and had assumed a character similar to a Greek gymnasium. Romans valued a suntan, as they would bathe nude, the suntan would also be seamless: *"Before taking their early afternoon bath, Romans would sunbathe under a portico or on a south-facing terrace thus gaining a fashionable tan. Since sunburn was associated with soldiers and people who lived in the countryside, a healthy tan gave the face a virile austerity that was liked by both aristocratic senators and former soldiers. A pallid complexion, on the other hand, seemed to bespeak the kind of man who spent his life indoors, banqueting and courting women, and who were therefore effeminate."* [40]

By 300 CE in the reign of Augustus, bathhouses often had separate facilities for women and men but this was not consistent. In different periods bathing was either mixed or single sex but was enjoyed nude. Various emperors forbade mixed bathing but the Romans did not always obey, periods of mixed nude bathing being well documented. In a period when mixed bathing was not allowed, a typical bath house would be open to men in the morning, women in the afternoon as the women were seen as second class. The morning was considered the best time to bathe.

The point is that public nudity in Roman times was not exceptional. Some Emperors would forbid mixed nude bathing but there were extended periods where such bathing was common place and quite normal. As with rulers down the centuries, power was the only consideration for them, if the people were enjoying themselves a bit too much, they felt they must act in order to exert their power. It was not in an effort to control sexual activity, that went on all time, it was to exercise power, to show the people who was boss. Hitler did much the same thing in the 1930s, non-National Socialist organisations were banned.

The Christians who lived and worked under Roman rule also bathed as the Romans did. One was a respected teacher, Clement. He fled to Antioch and then Jerusalem to avoid the persecution by Septimius Severus and died around 215 CE. In his work "The Educator", he wrote: *"There are, then, four reasons for the bath (for from that point I digressed in my oration), for which we frequent it: for cleanliness, or heat, or health, or lastly, for pleasure. Bathing for pleasure is to be omitted. For unblushing pleasure must be cut out by the roots; and the bath is to be taken by women for cleanliness and health, by men for health alone."* [41] Here we see the beginnings of what was to become commonplace in Christian thought, pleasure was sinful. These Christian teachers, far from simply teaching ideology, would recommend the use of power, *"... must be cut out by the roots"*. Force, not influence.

There were times when Christians participated in mixed bathing. *"During the dawning years of Christianity, before the decline of Rome, it was forbidden to bathe on Sundays and holidays, but before then the thermae were rarely closed for any reason. Sometimes men and women bathed together, but this custom varied from one period to another and depended upon local attitudes. At Pompeii and Badenweiler, for example, men and women bathed separately."* [42]

There is plenty of evidence that early Christians partook of mixed nude bathing. As Roy Bowen Ward says. "It is clear from Clement that in Alexandria at the end of the second century - contemporaneous with Irenaeus and Tertullian - mixed bathing by all classes was not only customary but also a popular activity in which Christian men and women engaged. [43]

It seems the indifference to nudity in Roman public life was shared by the earliest Christians. The story of Adam and Eve then makes sense if it is taken as one of deception rather than shameful nudity. Nude sculpture was found everywhere at the time.

The naked form was highly thought of in Roman society, not an attitude that would have resulted from a prudish view of nudity. I am not saying the Romans and Christians went nude everywhere nor that clothing had no importance. The point to note is simply that nudity at an appropriate place was not an issue, they did not fear nudity as do many in western societies today.

Christians against sex and nudity

After two centuries of persecution, Christianity was widespread throughout the Roman world but by about the third century, a cloud of darkness was spreading across the Christian world. Very slowly an anti-sex view point permeated the Christian movement. Nudity and sex were then seen as the same thing and became surrounded by moralistic platitudes. The ceremony of baptism, until then carried out nude, altered beyond recognition.

"We have to admit there is an immeasurable distance between all we read in the Bible and the practice of Christians." - Jacques Ellul [44] It is important to realise that anti-nudity attitudes did not come from the core teaching of Christians, they came from a small number of people. In historical terms, it is a mistake to judge figures from the past using modern values, but we would now see these people as damaged or even perverted. As Reay Tannahill says, "What the modern world still understands by "sin" stems not from the teaching of Jesus of Nazareth, or from the tablets handed down from Sinai, but from the early sexual vicissitudes of a handful of men who lived in the twilight days of imperial Rome" [45] As with any religious or political views, not everyone agreed or observed the "rules". There remained pockets of resistance to the anti-sex teachings. Sisinnius, Patriarch of Constantinople who died in 427 CE, still visited his local baths to bathe. When asked why he bathed twice a day, he said it was because bathing three times was inconvenient!

The anti-sex views were reaching previously unheard of heights of silliness. About this time, people like Emperor Licinius were making laws that prevented women and men from worshipping together. One man went so far as to request castration to prove his purity. He petitioned the Augustal Prefect for approval for the operation during the time of Justin Martyr (100-165 CE). Even though simple nudity has no direct link to sex, some Christians saw it differently. Following the Edict of Milan in 313 CE in the time of Emperor Constantine, Christianity became installed as the imperial religion of Rome and the great denial of human sexuality began in earnest. In 393 CE, the Olympic Games were banned because they were considered to be Pagan.

The classic story in the bible tells of the sin in the Garden of Eden. Here Adam and Eve succumbed to temptation. They ate of the forbidden fruit of the Tree of the Knowledge of Good and Evil and were subsequently cast out of the garden. They "knew they were naked", they felt shame and had to cover themselves. Until their sin, they would have been nude in the garden, supposedly free of sin, shame or temptation. Sex would have been seen as good and natural. It was only when they disobeyed and ate the forbidden fruit that they discovered "the knowledge". This knowledge we are told is that bodies were made unwholesome by their sin, not just that sex was bad, but our bodies are themselves bad.

This passage of the bible has generated all sorts of debate over its meaning, even a modest attempt at research yields a huge number of interpretations. Christian naturists will interpret it one way, right wing Christians will take it to mean that bodies are shameful. Genesis 3:7: says *"Then the eyes of both [Adam and Eve] were opened and they realised that they were naked; so they sewed fig leaves together and made coverings for themselves."* but in Genesis 1:31 it says *"And God saw everything that he had made, and, behold, [it was] very good."* These passages are interpreted in a large number of ways, one view assures us that nudity is shameful, another that nudity is pure and natural, all from the same text. The problem is at least partly due to the translation. It is unclear if the Hebrew text in the book of Genesis uses the word eromim translated as naked or arumim which means the uncovering of deceptions. The lack of clarity is because eromim and arumim appear the same in the Hebrew text. Genesis and the rest of the Torah was written using only consonants, with no letters to represent vowels. The key point to note is the view of the translator, if he was taught that nudity was shameful, he would of course use that as the translation, disregarding the fact that it makes a logical nonsense of the Adam and Eve story. There are also problems with the Hebrew word *chagowr*, translated above as *coverings*. This is usually taken to mean a belt for the waist, an apron. It comes from the Greek simikinthion and Latin semicinctium, meaning a half-girding or narrow covering. This translation would support the idea of nudity being shameful, an apron would cover genitals but Eve of course would still show her breasts. In Acts 19:12, chagowr refers to a wide belt or half-girdle worn by servants to protect clothing. Translators over the years have ascribed different meanings to chagowr. In the King James and Revised Standard Versions the meaning is taken as aprons which may have covered most of the body, the New American Standard Bible translates chagowr as loin coverings. but the Modern Language version gives skirts. The Living Bible says they covered themselves around the hip. The least specific is the New International Version which only uses the word coverings.

The story is about sin, Adam and Eve were told not to eat the forbidden fruit, they did eat and then tried to cover it up, to deceive. When they "made coverings for themselves" it makes sense to assume they did so to hide their deception rather than their nakedness. The prohibition was on eating the fruit, the sin was disobedience, trying to get away with it was proof of deception. It is their behaviour that is shameful rather than their genitals.

There are a whole range of opinions in between that take the same text and that comes to completely different conclusions. As above, this is partly due to problems with translation, but there is also the problem of words changing their meaning over time; awful once meant "full of awe", now it means only something truly bad. The argument will probably never be resolved and in all likelihood will get worse as the words in the bible have been translated into many differing languages, the speakers of each of these languages will come to yet more interpretations and these will themselves evolve and change. Some translations are difficult to accomplish so reliance is placed on earlier translations in other languages. Even the first English language versions of the Bible suffered from this problem, Miles Coverdale, credited with the first full printed version in English relied in part on William Tyndale's 16th

Century hand written version. Bible believers must place a great deal of trust in the linguistic skills of the translator.

Quite apart from augments over the meaning of "nakedness" in the story of Adam and Eve, the story continues when God says to Eve after being cast out of the Garden of Eden, *"I will greatly multiply thy sorrow and thy conception; in sorrow thou shalt bring forth children; and thy desire shall be to thy husband and he shall rule over thee"*. It is quite clear that this part of the bible was written by a man. Right from the start, women were looked down on by men, the story claims it was because Eve committed the first sin but really it was because a man wrote the book who was himself embedded in a social culture of male dominance. I find it interesting to note that Islam takes a pragmatic view over the problem of translation. The Quran is not considered the word of Allah except in the original Arabic. Translators are not trusted to get the meaning right.

The teachings of the bible have been extended and changed over the years. Men like Saint Maximos the Confessor or Saint Gregory of Nyssa, taught that the "chitones" or garments of skin showed the animal-like nature of people. Their cure for this ill was virginity, they argued that we should all strive to be virgins. Perhaps it did not occur to them but for rather obvious reasons, all the sects that follow this stricture to the letter, will die out!

A leading theologian of the fourth century, Saint Augustine, set the seal on the anti-sex teachings. He left his wife, illegitimate son and second mistress and turned his home in Hippo into a monastery. He considered sex a necessary evil, something not to be enjoyed, but a cold dutiful and mechanical act to be completed without passion. *"Perish the thought, that there should have been any unregulated excitement, or any excitement so great that they would ever need to resist desire!"* [46] From the modern view, it is interesting to note that he accepted violence as a legitimate means to force his views on others. *"It is indeed better (as no one ever could deny) that men should be led to worship God by teaching, than that they should be driven to it by fear of punishment or pain; but it does not follow that because the former course produces the better men, therefore those who do not yield to it should be neglected. For many have found advantage (as we have proved, and are daily proving by actual experiment), in being first compelled by fear or pain, so that they might afterwards be influenced by teaching, or might follow out in act what they had already learned in word."* [47] The Order of St. Augustine of course say he only preached peace, love and goodwill to all. Sadly this did not include women. As St. Augustine said, *"Women should not be enlightened or educated in any way. They should, in fact, be segregated as they are the cause of hideous and involuntary erections in holy men.".* This idea is prevalent in the Taliban even today.

Arnobius (317 CE) called intercourse "filthy and degrading", and that it is blasphemous to say that Jesus *"was born of vile coitus and came into the light as a result of the spewing forth of senseless semen, a product of obscene gropings".* Others followed in a similar manner including Methodius and Ambrose. Saint John Chrysostom said *"Among all savage beasts, none is found as harmful as woman.".* Tertullian taught that sexual intercourse drives out the Holy Spirit and that women were "the devil's door: through them Satan creeps into men's hearts and minds and works his wiles for their spiritual destruction."

By the eighth century a very strict set of anti-sex rules and penalties was in place, refusal to comply meant punishment on earth and the possibility of eternity in hell. Women were sinful and were guilty of tempting men; if they succumbed, the women were the more guilty. God was seen as the forgiver of sins, peace in the next world gained by pain in this. All this gave Christians a great problem, not only the means by which Mary became pregnant, but how she gave birth without the baby touching her Pudendum, her part of shame. All sorts of means were suggested to explain how it happened, some saying that Jesus emerged through Mary's breast or navel, others that he descended from Heaven fully formed, thus avoiding the whole question. The pubic area of a women has been known for a long time as the

Pudendum. The word is from the Latin root "pudo", the verb meaning to be ashamed or *"that of which one ought to be or to feel ashamed or, indeed, ashamed to mention"*.

The so-called fig-leaf campaign was pursued by the Roman Catholic Church, its aim was to cover all nudity in art. In October 1541 Michelangelo finished the "Last Judgment" but was accused of "intolerable obscenity" during the fig-leaf campaign for his nude depictions showing genitals. Cardinal Carafa and Monsignor Sernini campaigned to remove the frescoes, but the Pope resisted. This is interesting as the work was inside his private chapel. On Michelangelo's death, a law was issued to cover genitals. [48]

This resulted in Michelangelo's apprentice, Daniele da Volterra, covering the genitals with perizomas or briefs. Restoration work carried out in 1993 left the perizomas in place but a faithful uncensored copy of the original by Marcello Venusti can be seen at the Capodimonte Museum in Naples. Other works fell foul of the fig-leaf campaign such as the bronze statue of Cristo della Minerva [49] and the statue of the naked child Jesus in "Madonna of Bruges" (Belgium).

Even though sex was seen as loathsome and only required for procreation, the real sin was the experience of sexual pleasure. Marital sex was supposed to be limited to procreation and enjoyment limited as far as possible. The more extreme advocated a sheet or animal skin with a hole cut in for the penis to minimise any pleasure. Not every Christian teacher followed this, Saint Paul insisted that couples should not "defraud" each other of their sexual rights, they belonged to each other. Such extreme views are not core teachings but the view of a few unfortunate people. Perhaps the Catholic Church is changing, Pope John Paul II is widely quoted as saying *"The human body can remain nude and uncovered and preserve its splendour and its beauty."* He also said *"Sexual modesty cannot in any simple way be identified with the use of clothing, nor shamelessness with the absence of clothing and total or partial nakedness. There are circumstances in which nakedness is not immodest. Nakedness, as such, is not to be equated with physical shamelessness. Immodesty is present only when nakedness plays a negative role with regards to the value of the person... The human body is not in itself shameful, nor for the same reason are sensual reactions, and human sensuality in general. Shamelessness (just like shame and modesty) is a function of the interior of the person."*

Suppressed sexuality manifested itself in appalling practices, some of them elevated to a virtue. These include flagellation of penitents, self-mutilation, castration, witch-hunts and religious massacres. Some religious sects still value Corporal Mortification, flagellation as being more important than sex, a gross perversion of human nature. *"No one can ever quantify the mental anguish inflicted upon Christian believers through the centuries, an anguish beyond comprehension of other people; accepting in their minds [as] divine truths that every fibre of their body impelled them to ignore, they were forever haunted by fear of the fires of hell and thereby even suffered the torments of the damned during their life on earth"* [50]

In 1428, the Bishop of Lincoln led a large procession to the Church of St. Mary, Lutterworth. There he presided over the exhumation, denunciation and burning of the body of John Wycliffe, a man who had made the first translation of the bible into English a little over 40 years earlier. His work was condemned as heresy. This is an excellent example of the means by which Christianity was spread whilst retaining power in the hands of a few. Only the priests and a small number of scholars were able to read the bible and people had to trust their interpretation. As interpretation of the bible is at the very least, controversial, the trust placed in these often damaged individuals was too great but it enabled them to retain power. It was they who defined who were good and who were not and the people believed them, after all, they were the learned ones, those who knew the Word of God. This first English translation predated printing so was laboriously hand copied, a fact which limited its circulation but for the first time, many more could read its message. There were an enormous number who could not read at all so could not benefit and it took more than another century for printed versions of the Bible in English became available, but the grip the priests had held for so long was weakened. The power of the Catholic Church was challenged in England by Henry VIIIth who saw the Bible in English as a strong political counter to the power of Rome. William Tyndale, later burned as a heretic, brought out an incomplete printed English version but the first full English version of was produced in 1535 by Miles Coverdale. He relied on Tyndale's translation for the New Testament and parts of the Old Testament, for the rest he used amongst other sources, Martin Luther's German Bible.

A flood of translations followed amongst them the Geneva Bible of 1560 and the King James Bible of 1611. Helped by these, England changed from the most pro-Catholic country in Europe to the most virulently anti-Catholic.

Even today some Christian churches still teach that sex is for procreation only, not for pleasure. How many of their parishioners appreciate that these views come not from the bible nor from the teachings of Jesus, but from a small number of individuals who by measures of their times were abnormal but from a modern view were damaged individuals. The way this relates to social nudity is clear, those who would teach that sex is bad will also teach that nudity is bad on the grounds that one causes the other. They have no evidence for this, they simply conform to their memes. In an act of pure madness, the town of Villahermosa in Mexico passed a law banning indoor nudity, not in some long passed prudish era but on 22nd December 2004. It is very hard to imagine how this law is to be policed but offenders face 36 hours in jail or a fine of US$120. Mexico is a stronghold of the Catholic church.

Programmes such as the Moral Maze broadcast on the BBC often show there will never be an absolute morality for all to follow, what is preached by one group as immoral is encouraged by others. It is easy to construct moral dilemmas that are not easy to answer. The important point surely is to live without hurting others, simple nudity cannot hurt other people.

Dilemmas

Liberty means responsibility. That is why most men dread it.
George Bernard Shaw

Should I be free to be naked?

Should I be free to be naked in the company of other people who do not choose to be naturists? What should I do when a visitor comes to my house? I feel that I should be free to dress or not as I choose, however, I am acutely aware of the sensitivity others show on the subject of nudity. A balance must be struck but it leads to a more interesting question, if I dress when they visit my house in order to suit their sensibilities, should not they undress when I visit their house, in order to suit mine? On the face of it, it seems a fair question.

To extend the idea, suppose I call into question aspects of other people's lifestyles that do not accord with my view of the world. Many would be offended or at the very least, disagree with me. For example, should I try to deny an aspect of someone's belief in a religion if I do not share their belief? Believers consider it their right to believe, and I happen to agree with them so it is clear I should not challenge them. Now consider their attitude to my belief that naturism is a healthy way of life, one that promotes respect and tolerance for others. Should I have my beliefs cast out as being unworthy or is the right to hold an honest belief only reserved for members of large religious groups?

If we are to have an equitable world, there must be room for everyone's beliefs unless those beliefs cause harm to others; it is very difficult to imagine how naturism can harm anyone. Saying that I should never be naked in my garden on the grounds that I may be seen and offend others is like asking a Christian nun in her habit to be always hidden from view. Her habit is a mark of her beliefs and she would claim the right to hold those beliefs and to use her habit as her witness. Tolerance is what is required, tolerance of other people's beliefs and values, even if they do not accord with your own. Naturism is not a threat to others so why some fear nudity and take strong action against nude people is hard to understand. Perhaps they think freedom of thought only applies to their religion. Like the first Ford cars, you can have what colour you like as long as its black. Study of any aspect of human society shows there is always a wide spread of belief no matter how hard some will try to unify ideas. Naturism has a rightful place in society and has taken its place amongst all the other ideas clamouring for attention, all I ask is that I am not persecuted nor ridiculed.

Should social nudity be banned on the grounds of aesthetics? Should anyone overweight, unattractive and all men be forever forced to be naked only in the shower? This is an extremely dangerous argument. Imagine if only the "beautiful people" can be naked, with the rest of us that do not conform to a standard being forced to cover up. This is very close to the ideas pursued by the fascists, they considered the Aryan race were the pinnacle of the human form, all others being lesser beings. In our spin and image conscious world, many people fear their body does not look sufficiently attractive; they fear it does not measure up to the perfection of the fashion industry.

It is very clear that looks have nothing to do with naturism. Your body is what it is, accepting that body as it is leads to a far happier life. All the research into self-image or self-worth shows that naturists have a far better image of themselves and consequently suffer less from some of the modern social ills. [51]

Being seen by others

What happens if I am working naked at home and someone sees me from their house across the road? If they have nothing better to do than spy on other people, they should accept they may see things they would otherwise choose not to. On the other hand, if I were to "parade in front of the window" that would be a very different issue. In any case, I would argue that is not naturism, it is exhibitionism and is not what makes life pleasant for me. As in many aspects of life, a balance must be made. I often sit naked working at my computer; in theory someone across the road could see in although they would not be able to see very much. It does not concern me if they know I am not dressed, as long as nothing I do could be considered offensive.

Sitting typing this text can hardly be offensive! The same applies if I am doing the vacuum cleaning or tidying up etc. Should I draw the curtains first? To me that is not a sensible course of action as there is nothing shameful about simply being naked. Usually I glance out of the window and check to see if anyone may be directly outside. As there usually is not, I continue with my job as normal. If someone was there, I just wait a moment for them to move on simply to avoid upsetting them as good manners, but I also recognise my right to my lifestyle.

If I sit in my garden and have made reasonably sure I am in a secluded place, what should I do if someone climbs on a fence and sees me, especially if a child does the climbing? If this happens, as it did one summer, I wait until the person goes away then retire into the house. I am not concerned about people seeing me nude, nudity is not an issue, but I do care about upsetting people. When they realise there is nothing special going on, they lose interest and go away. I should not need to construct special arrangements to prevent any possible view of my garden, reasonable care is all that is required. If they climb a fence to gain a view, they should not be surprised if they see something they may not appreciate!

Art

The nude in art has little or nothing to do with naturism. In the art world, a clear distinction is drawn between the naked and the nude. Much is written about this distinction and about how it has changed over time. In past centuries, images of the nude were acceptable because they portrayed perfection, an idealised view of a compliant woman. Paintings were a status symbol, including those of the nude. Only the very rich could afford them. We now look at them in galleries or as copies in books so they are taken out of context. They were painted to be hung in churches and private houses to be viewed by the owner and shown to guests to impress them. They were a demonstration of the wealth and by inference, the power of men.

In Eastern culture, paintings that were intended to convey sexuality showed an explicit sexual act, usually with the woman taking an equal role to the man. They conveyed the pleasure to be had by sex. In the European tradition, the nude played a different role, the women were nude, serene and above all, passive to the more powerful viewer, always assumed to be men. They were more statements of power than sensuality. Those who painted outside of this tradition were shunned by the establishment. It took a complete social revolution to change the status quo.

Image and Spin

The modern world seems very keen on image. There are numerous TV programmes that focus on image, mostly concentrating on how to achieve a given look. One could be forgiven if people watching got the idea that looks are everything, that it does not matter what you feel inside, how you behave, as long as you appear to fit into a specific social set. Whilst much of this is quite harmless, some use fashion as a shield, they hide their true personality behind a façade. The dark side of this behaviour is why they do it, what are they hiding? If people spend much of their lives pursuing an image, they are in danger of living an empty, vacuous existence. In contrast, naturists can hardly be pursuing an image. People are judged instead by their behaviour, what kind of people they really are.

This interest in image seems to be common at every level in society. In recent years, political parties and governments have pursued their image at the cost of discarding their principles. Specialist advisors are employed to give a spin to each communication, to create a false impression of what is actually happening or about to happen.

I would argue in favour of honesty, to say what is in your heart as truly as the limitations of language will allow. Although there is no absolute measure of truth, what is important is the intention to be as true as possible. In declaring my belief that social nudity is a healthy lifestyle, I am saying it from as truthful a point of view as I am able. This declaration does not accord with a desire to achieve an image, I desire instead to be myself. If a dishonest person dresses to create a given impression, it is easier to be taken in than if they are not trying to achieve that image. I always remember that Hitler wore a suit.

Naturist Controversies

As with all human activity, there are controversies amongst naturists. The most common, the argument over the words nudist and naturist is also the most trivial. As Bill Bryson says in his excellent book Mother Tongue, no one controls English, it changes over time all by itself. Attempts to control language such as those by the Institute Francais with the French language, always fail. Those who try to enforce a definition on the words nudist or naturist are missing the point, the words mean whatever they mean to "the many", not just those interested in leading a nude life. If most of the population take the two words as synonymous, there is nothing that can be done about it!

Some naturist clubs in the UK will not allow members to be tattooed, have their pubic hair shaved or be pierced. For a club formed by people who themselves have been victims of repression, it is odd they repress the lifestyle of others.

Sex and naturism

Human sexuality is a huge subject and I have no intention of attempting to cover it here, but the connection between sexual behaviour and naturism is clearly of importance. Much has been written about naturism, most states explicitly that naturism is not sexual. This is true but needs some explanation. It is more accurate to say that naturism is not overtly sexual, that is to say, the experience of a socially nude environment is not stimulating in a direct or simple manner. Naturists have sex, there is nothing celibate about naturists but it is a result of normal human relationships, not as a result of their naturism.

Being nude has a strong sensual element, for many this is the main reason they lead such a lifestyle and connection between sensual and sexual experience is easy to see, but one does not necessarily lead to the other. One can lead to the other if you desire it to, just as an intimate dinner for two can lead to sex, but the desire must be there in the first place.

Just as no one would claim that every meal is a precursor to sex, I would claim that the experience of social nudity is not a precursor to sex. One does not cause the other, nudity leads first and foremost to sensual enjoyment. If that later leads to a sexual encounter then that is fine, but the connection is not automatic.

I like to think of sexuality and sensuality as being connected by a line, a continuum of feelings that slowly changes from one end to the other. Some activities are either explicitly sexual at one end or clearly sensual at the other. Other activities come somewhere in between, like the use of massage oils in the foreplay before lovemaking. I contend that naturism is firmly at the sensual end of this line.

As Werner Zimmermann said in his early work on naturism, *"Nudism is unerotic in itself though some individuals may be led to it by their erotic needs. The body becomes quite natural; it is no longer perceived in sexual terms. The physical attributes of sex no longer play a special role. They are simply there, like the nose or the mouth. Accordingly, the naked life in itself cannot offer any particular erotic gratification or relief to a mature person. It may well largely eliminate the over stimulation of the sexual instinct, but not the instinct itself! Nor is it meant to! The mature human being without sexual power, without generative power, without creative power, would be an unnatural, pitiable cripple!"* [52]

Women, myths and naturism

There is a myth that men find naturism more attractive than women. This results from asking the wrong question because experience demonstrates that women enjoy naturism just as much as men. Some naturist establishments have a gender imbalance with more men than women. A visit to le Cap d'Agde will provide ample evidence, there you will find about equal numbers of men and women, mainly as families, couples and a few singles. It is important to understand why some naturist places do have a gender imbalance. The problem is not that women do not or would not enjoy a nude lifestyle, quite the opposite, but something powerful holds them back.

So what holds women back? There are several problems described by women and their friends, namely:

- Dissatisfaction with body size or shape

- Cultural disapproval of nudity in general

- Fear of assault or sexual harassment

- Fear of being a target of voyeurism

- Too few other women to socialise with

Body size or shape

Many feel they have less than perfect bodies and that staying dressed enables them to hide it away. This hunt for the body beautiful is driven by magazines, the fashion trade, celebrities and the modern trend of valuing presentation over content. Men are less prone to this belief so are more likely to take up a naturist lifestyle, they care less about their image.

It is common to meet people who are happy to admit they would not be seen dead in that colour or that dress. Sadly, these people feel comforted by conforming to a fashion set for them by those who make money out of them. Who actually decides what colour or style is in this year or this season? Is the style ever the same for two years running? Of course not, the business interests that force fashion change would not make so much money.

Realising that the fashion industry is manipulative is the first step, the second step is to decide what should be done about it.

Taking up a nude lifestyle will never be for everyone, it would be daft to promote such an idea, but a such a lifestyle is a viable option and should be treated as such, one way to live without harming other people. Only a small percentage of the population, either men or women, come close to matching the images set out by the fashion industry. Failure to accept this mostly leads to misery. Occasionally there is the contrasting position. In an effort to sell more clothes to those who were not the same size and shape as fashion models, Marks and Spencers used an advert that featured a nude women in a hill, declaring *"I'm normal"*. She was not a supermodel but a normal person one would meet anywhere.

Having shed the need for fashion, one can retain clothes but feel more freedom, freedom from being manipulated. Once women also realise that in a naturist environment, it really really does not matter what size or shape you are, the sense of relief, the sense of freedom can be most rewarding. The naturist women I know are more confident in their outlook, they accept their bodies and those of other people and as a result, are happier. Those infatuated with clothes use them as a status symbol to hide behind. When you are naked, you are what you are, there is no need to hide.

How much misery has been cause to those who feel the need to diet to lose weight, not for health reasons but to conform to the latest body size standard? Many women have suffered greatly to achieve this, anorexia and bulimia being distressingly common. Some will have surgery for breast enhancement, others for breast reduction, there is liposuction, botox and a whole range of very lucrative so called body enhancements.

By far the largest number of magazines are aimed at women and a large measure of their content is based on fashion and make-up. The magazines must sell well or they would be off the shelves. This indicates that large numbers of women are keen to conform to the latest fashion. Why should this be such a preoccupation? Wearing the latest fashion allows one to blend in with others, to be part of the scene.

The very best body enhancement technique is to come to terms with one's body. It does wonders for self-confidence, being able to say to one's self *"I don't care about my cellulite or my breasts heading south, this is ME"*.

In France, Austria, Germany and other countries where nakedness is well accepted, they have far less of a problem with "Essex Man" and "Essex Girl", those who live a vacuous, image driven life. These people have a poor self-image but try to achieve self-confidence with the "right" clothes, cars and makeup. They could not consider being seen in public unless they had their tribal clothing in place. People who deep down have a poor self-image, also cover up by becoming judgmental of others. They always wear the right clothing for each occasion so they won't be judged badly. Naturism is far more open, you are what you are.

Cultural disapproval of nudity in general

It can be hard to "admit" a desire to be socially nude, some will misinterpret the motive. The experience of a great majority of people who have come out and talked openly of their interests in naturism has been very positive. Some have been met with bemused responses but most are either neutral or even encouraging. Others may not want to take part but are happy to acknowledge it in others.

Fear of assault or sexual harassment

The rate of crime in general and of sex related crime in particular is lower in naturist environments. It is not easy to point to the reason for this except of course that people more at ease with their bodies are less likely to commit sex related crime. The worst of these crimes occur in the always dressed world, people known to naturists as textiles.

Most sex attacks are perpetrated by those known to the victim, rape is more commonly committed by acquaintances or even family members than by strangers. A naturist environment will not protect against these predators but at least a sexually excited man is easier to spot!

Rape is a crime of violence, the projection of power over another usually weaker victim, the sexual aspect is secondary to the grave act of violence. Crime does occur in naturist areas, there is nowhere on earth free of such behaviour, but naturism does not encourage it nor does it cause it.

One advantage of naturism often promoted by naturism is its social nature, the friendliness. In friendly social groups there is support from others, even safety in numbers. The accusation of sexual harassment is taken very seriously by naturists and those that run the clubs and resorts, any such deviant behaviour is dealt with very quickly.

It is normally judged that women are safer in a naturist environment, more from the self-selecting group of people there than any set of rules or means of enforcement.

Fear of being a target of voyeurism

Do naturists look at other nude people? Of course they do, just like at any pavement café, people watch other people but that does not mean they gawp, stare or look with lewd intention. There is a huge difference between admiring a naked person and lusting after them, the difference lies in your heart not in your eyes.

Women are taught from an early age to cover up, to hide themselves from the unwanted gaze of men. After years of such teaching, it is not hard to understand why taking clothes off in a public setting is harder for women. In contrast, many women like to be admired, as with most things in life, there is no one fits all, some like being seen nude, some don't. Experience shows that in socially nude places, people do not stare and look no more than in another social gathering.

A non-naturist may feel that when they are naked, they will become the centre of attention. This may happen of you stripped off in the local supermarket but not when everyone else is naked. This has even come as a slight shock, after having wrestled for years with their attitude to stripping off and having actually done it, nothing happens. No-one takes any notice at all.

Too few other women to socialise with

The final problem is self-perpetuating, that if there are more men at a naturist club, there "must" be some reason for it so women will not go. There is no reason, so if the circle is broken, this problem will disappear. Gender imbalance is a symptom, not the underlying problem.

Some naturist clubs enforce a gender balance but the same mind-set that enforces the balance also forces other "rules" that many find oppressive. No wonder such places are in serious decline. Women like to socialise with other women so having a gender imbalance is not likely to encourage new women naturists.

What is needed is to move away from the old club naturist model and towards more openness, have more naturist holiday resorts and swims. In the UK some local authorities are approaching naturist clubs to run such swimming events.

There are more and more naturist or clothes optional resorts opening around the world, all very welcome developments that will help women in particular to enjoy a clothes free life, even if only for a short while.

Men, myths and naturism

Another myth is that men take up naturism for sexual reasons, perhaps they are voyeurs, exhibitionists or just plain perverts. This myth is also easy to dispose of, a visit to any naturist place will show just how non-alluring a sea of naked bodies can be. A question often asked about naturism is about erections. Experience shows that is not a problem, it doesn't happen, why should they in a non-sexual environment? If a man did go to a naturist place for sexual reasons, he would be easy to spot!

It is true that occasional voyeurs can be seen hiding in the dunes behind some nude beaches, but these are not those who espouse a naturist lifestyle.

They are easy to spot, they have shy, embarrassed faces, binoculars and exhibit a bobbing up and down manner akin to meer cats. Indeed this is the name often given to these sad people. They are not naturists in the sense meant in this book, they do not believe in the philosophy of naturism, that of a sense of freedom and body acceptance.

Media and the arts

Newspapers

In August 2004, a brief look at articles that refer to naturism published on the Guardian website [53] showed that most showed a neutral or positive attitude. The general tone was one of acceptance, naturism would be simply listed along with other activities. Kirsty Scott's article in August 2003 simply reported *"...naked rambler has vowed to continue the final leg of his naturist trail across the UK"*. No puns, just reporting just like Amanda Thompson's article, also August 2003, where she wrote *"Taking your clothes off in public is not something that comes easily to the British. You only have to hint at the word "nude" to have people blushing or sniggering like schoolchildren. But not naturists, who take their clothes off outdoors simply because they enjoy the freedom and the sensation of the sun and fresh air on their skin. Naked rambling, anyone?"*

Those articles written by journalists that have actually tried a socially nude environment all showed their surprise at how pleasant it was, even if they did not choose to go again. Luke Harding writing in September 2003 said *"I went for a final nude dip. The sky was grey and rainy. I dried in the communal changing rooms. I felt terrific."* David Atkinson wrote that "In short, if you're looking for an orgy, then you've come to the wrong place. And, if you adhere to concepts of body fascism or exhibitionism, then go elsewhere. Naturism is not for you."

One or two writers could not resist the old puns, old habits die hard. Perhaps they will learn from their peers; the days when taking the rise out of "cripples", "blacks" and "foreigners" have passed, so perhaps the use of pejorative terms about naturists is also dying out.

Some were negative, in June 2003, Stuart Jeffries reported on a newspaper stunt, he said *"In an attempt to restore some decency in these debauched times we invited Guardian readers to pose for our own Spencer Tunick-style artwork on Brighton beach yesterday."* What evidence has he that we live in "debauched times", is it the bombing of Iraq, supplying arms and other aid to oppressive governments? Probably not, that and similar has gone on for decades. No, his "evidence" is his own body loathing. He no doubt felt pleased with himself while he *"watched our award-winning photographer Eamonn McCabe strike a blow against the exhibitionists"*. As for decency, does running a stunt count as decent? Is creating news to sell papers a proper way to behave or should he stick to reporting what people actually do and think? One can infer what he thinks by the final part of his article when he concentrates on *"..other people's dingly danglies"*. Perhaps he doesn't have any.

Perhaps Catherine Bennett has a fair dose of body guilt herself. In April 2003 she wrote that *"even those who wonder what, other than seedy exhibitionism, might motivate those who wish to display themselves in this way."* Of course she misses the point, most people, myself included, do not go to naturist beaches to "display" anything, quite the opposite, many are happy if there is no one else there. If she had the courage to join with a group of naturists perhaps she would gain sufficient self-confidence to ignore ideas of "display" and simply accept her own body for what it is, no matter what shape or size. In May 2001 she wrote *"It's not every day, after all, that the disgusting act of nudity is perpetrated by a youngish blonde".* Her body guilt is plain to see, she sees nudity as "disgusting". It must be tricky for her to have a shower.

In June 1999, Jonathan Margolis wrote an article called "Dark side of fresh air Utopians" about H&E Naturist magazine. He makes a valid point about the early naturists, some of them seemed dangerously close to the fascist point of view, seeking after the perfect body as described in the section on the history of naturism. Sadly he misses the point about modern naturism. Once someone has got rid of their body guilt, nudity becomes ordinary but Margolis says *"But what puts the magazine into the bizarre category are the advertisements"*, *"One announces the services of a nude home cleaner and another of a naturist cabinet maker."* Well yes they would wouldn't they, it is a magazine that promotes nudity. He finds it bizarre because he failed to understand the naturist philosophy. I do not mean he did not want to join in, that is a matter of choice, but as a journalist he did not report when he saw, he reported his own prejudice.

Also advertised in the magazine were *"escort and massage services, suppliers of naturist videos and full-page ads for a film developing service."* I suppose there were, just as there are in all the newspapers I looked at, the free ones that rain through the door and those he writes for, so what is his point? He is implying that *"escort and massage services"* equate with prostitution, therefore naturists are prostitutes? Dogs like chocolate, you like chocolate, therefore you are dog. Free newspapers advertise *"escort and massage services"* so all readers of free newspapers either are prostitutes or use the services of prostitutes. A quite preposterous assertion. Also advertised were *"wholemeal bread, rupture belts, vitamin pills, bust enhancement products and penis extenders"*, again, just like almost every newspaper and many magazines. Later in the article he says *"H&E today looks like a bad soft porn mag."* Presumably he reads good and bad porn mags to make the comparison. Notice the cheap journalistic trick I have used here? It is in the same low class as *"have you stopped beating your wife, answer yes or no"*. Ignoring my cheap jibe, his point is quite good, many naturists have complained about the number of young professional female models in H&E and how that does not show "real" naturists.

He claims that *"The obsession with photography is powerful evidence that naturism has at least as much to do with voyeurism as with a philosophical belief in not wearing clothes."* Not at all, the large number of photographs sell magazines. That may or may not be naturism, but he cannot claim that naturism is about voyeurism, at least he gives no evidence for it.

Going on he makes a good point, *"Naturism's serious dubiousness lies in its roots. A reaction at the end of the 19th century to the stuffiness and hypocrisy of previous decades, it rapidly became a cult of the perfect body."* (....) *"By developing a culture of body fascism, were nudists moving towards real fascism? And even if they were, does that in any way pollute the naturism of today?"* (....) *"Early nudism was stirring stuff, with no smoking or drinking, and compulsory vegetarianism and callisthenics - the type of regime which George Orwell, with a keener eye than most intellectuals for nascent fascism, loathed."* and *"But the December 1939 H&E includes a glowing piece about how naturism was faring under Mussolini."*

But then he says *"Today's nudism, as reflected by H&E, is no longer fascist-inspired"*. A well-made point and quite true. But first asking about fascist influences in naturism then saying there are none in the modern movement is the same kind of trick used with photograph placement on a newspaper page or even the old *"have you stopped beating your wife"*. For example, if a headline that says *"Man acquitted of drink driving"* is placed in a column next to an unconnected photograph of a car crash, the implication is created that he was in fact guilty. This is a common though very cheap trick, not good journalism. Nowadays, far from promoting perfect bodies, naturism promotes body acceptance, it really does not matter what shape or size you are, you will be more likely to be accepted for what you are in naturist environment than in the fashion and image conscious one promoted at least in part by newspapers.

Then Margolis really ruins it all, he goes on to say *"It is a sense that readers are being invited to laugh at the uglier nudists; here are some good-looking models, here are some pudgy, bespectacled suburbanites: you choose."* Does he laugh at those who are overweight? Is being "bespectacled" funny? It sounds to me that he is the body fascist hiding behind a journalist smirk.

It is good to see that most Guardian articles were positive towards naturism, this is a great improvement on those of a decade ago or more when the nudge-nudge style was more prevalent. The tabloid press are somewhat different but then they are known to write anything that sells, lies, jibes and the plain silly. Don't buy them; the tabloid press is hardly worth a mention as their record in accurate reporting is very slim. Items in the tabloids might refer to the "size of his manhood" or "a big girl". The sick individuals who write this stuff are so inhibited they cannot even refer to body parts without using euphemisms. The size of a woman's breasts or the length of a man's penis has no effect at all on their worth as a human being but then the writer's job is to sell newspapers.

Television

There have been a good number of programmes on British television recently that portray naturism in a good light. The script writers cannot lose their old habits that easily so some of the clichés crop up, but on the whole the reporting is fair.

In contrast, a programme called "The World's Best Nude Beaches" shows the US media are a long way behind the Europeans when it comes to attitudes. This is shown clearly in a portion of the text on the website of the Travel Channel promoting programme. It says (the programme) *"The World's Best Nude Beaches" is good, (not entirely) clean fun. From the Caribbean to Europe to the U.S. and beyond, we'll discover where to go, what to do, and who to do it with - while letting it all hang out. Join us as we get just a little bit naughty on the World's Best Nude Beaches."* The actual programme had one of the worst voice over commentaries that has been broadcast in recent years. The writers took a great deal of trouble to include all the old double-entendres, clichés and misunderstandings. No wonder that on the website they used the phrase *"good, (not entirely) clean fun"*, there was no visual "dirt" on the programme, the dirt is in their minds and in the script. They demonstrate a genital obsession as is shown by writing "while letting it all hang out", missing the point that a naked man has nothing to hang out "of". As the programme is shown around the world, I wonder of the programme makers realise just how lame and old fashioned this style of writing has become?

Pornography

Although it is a large and important subject, pornography has no direct relevance to naturism except in the way that some nude images are wrongly treated as porn. Pornography and naturism are almost total opposites, porn treats people, especially women and children, as objects, pieces of meat that have certain body parts of interest to a certain class of viewer. In contrast, naturism fosters people as people, disregarding their shape and size. There have been people that have reported that they ended a long time search for perfect porn when they discovered the benefits of seeing others as people. Seeing beautiful nude images as pictures of people rather than sexual meat, their life changed.

A photograph of a nude can be porn, art, or simply a record. It depends on the viewer, the context of the picture and the skill of the image maker. The real difference lies in the intent of the image maker and that of the viewer. A close-up photograph of a woman's genitals could form a useful part of a medical book or as an image on a porn website. Doctors using the medical book to learn more about anatomy are hardly consumers of porn but would become such if their intent was sexual gratification. Law courts have found this aspect of porn very troublesome, it is simply not possible to define whether a particular image or set of images is pornographic or not. It is rather like the classic difference between a ship and a boat, everyone "knows" the difference yet cannot define it. Many pornographic publications are obvious for what they are, porn, but many are not. Customs officials still occasionally seize naturist magazines, failing to understand the difference. They fall foul of the tick box, if a certain number of their tick boxes say "porn", to them it is porn regardless of common sense.

Thankfully, the law courts are more in touch with common sense. A good example occurred in 1998, James and Carolyn Scarlett won an important legal case against HM Customs & Excise. They are the proprietors of a company that sells naturist videos, books etc. called Tower Productions. The Customs had arrested them under the Protection of Children Act (1978) for importing and distributing naturist books and videos. They were released without charges being made but a Destruction Order was made on material such as the video La Borde, Richard West's Canada Naturally - The Book, and one of Tower's own productions A Naturist's Provence - Part Two. Copies of the book Elizabeth's Dream by Julia Free Hand were also due to be destroyed. It seems the problem that the Customs people focused on was indecent pictures of children but on the 7th July, the Cheltenham Magistrates Court did not agree with HM Customs & Excise. The Scarletts were awarded £1,400 costs and the court ordered the return of the material.

In the end, I find porn is boring as it has nothing of value, it is just a commodity produced and consumed by those who know the cost of everything but the value of nothing. It is said that porn devalues women. That is true but it devalues the consumer much more.

For a long time people have argued over the meaning of words. Most of the arguments are fruitless because meanings evolve, they are not fixed by committees, authorities or august bodies of experts. Perhaps the most common word to cause argument is the word "art". A particular piece of work will cause people to ask *"is it art?"* This invariably results in the formation of at least two groups who then use all their power and passion to convince others of the rightness of their cause.

Minds do not meet, no advance is made. Another word that causes such schism is pornography. The groups that result from the inevitable argument disagree as they would over art but with much greater passion. Not long into the debate, one set of arguments will be justified by the belief that others will be protected from harm but the ones that pursue this line have not required this protection themselves. They have gone through life and come out as well rounded, sensible people free from the bad effects of pornography. In quick time, the special case of children will be introduced and henceforth, all reason lost in the ensuing maelstrom of passion.

Before the Victorian era, pornography in its modern sense did not exist. Humans have been depicting sexual scenes for centuries but it was only in the 19th Century that such scenes were described as pornography. It took the zeal of the Victorians to popularise a specific word to describe the depiction of sex, they saw all sexually explicit images as A Bad Thing. Some use it to mean anything showing nudity, others to mean the depiction of sexual activity, still others will only use the word to describe hard core sex. The word itself is old, from arcane Greek but first appeared in an English medical dictionary in 1857.

Its meaning was neutral and referred to the literature and images that surrounded the mounting problem of prostitution in Victorian England. Once "re-invented", within 5 years of its first appearance in England, the American lexicographer Webster [Noah Webster (1758-1843) American lexicographer] added it to his dictionary, but in line with his moralising habit, added a new meaning.

The Collins Dictionary defines pornography as *"...writings, pictures, films etc. designed to stimulate sexual excitement"*, the word coming from the Greek word pornographos, the writings of harlots."* As a comparison, the same dictionary defines the word erotic as *"...arousing sexual desire or giving sexual pleasure"* and the word erotica is defined as *"explicitly sexual material or art"*, both words having the Greek word eros as a base, i.e. love.

The problem with these definitions is the lack of clarity between them, both are concerned with sexual arousal but erotic seems to imply love and pleasure whereas pornography implies cheap excitement. If this is so, pornography would be seen by some as sinful whereas something that was simply erotic would be acceptable. In the eyes of some religious thinkers, eroticism would be acceptable, even desirable, inside of a married relationship.

The discovery of the lost city of Pompeii in the mid 18th Century was greeted with great enthusiasm. This was however damped when it was discovered that many of the images and sculptures depicted sexual activity. [54] None were hidden, they were found in rooms that were used for everyday family life including those where visitors would be welcomed.

With post Victorian sensibilities it is hard to imagine a social environment where sexual images were all around but the fact is, the Romans saw sex and its depiction in a quite different way. They had their taboos but these were more to do with who one had sex with rather than the sex itself. It would be socially unacceptable for a master to have sex with a servant but servants and their masters would consider sex and its depiction quite normal and not something to be hidden away.

Some of the archaeologists of the time defaced what they found but in doing so, drew more attention than ever. They had failed to realise that the Romans thought that not to have sexual pictures showed that you did not have taste and did not understand your society. [55]

The movable art works of a sexual nature were removed to the Museo Borbonico near Naples, where a secret museum was established. Only influential males could get access and then only after a rigorous selection process. The most famous item is a sculpture of the God Pan having sex with a goat. The quality of the carving and the general execution of the piece indicates that it was not an item for a cheap thrill in the manner of modern porn, it was an piece that would have been on display for all to see. Most likely it would have a strong cultural meaning for the owner but also been seen as humorous. It would not have been seen from the modern view, an act so hideous that many even now think is more serious than murder.

The Victorians thought that viewing sexually explicit art work corrupted the weak, specifically women, children and the working classes. The law makers naturally thought of themselves as being immune to this corrupting effect, they were from the social class allowed access to the secret museum in Naples and the one brought into existence in the British Museum. They thought that anything that weakened the lower classes would prevent them from working so should be avoided at all costs. In their view, sexually explicit images cause sexual perversion and "self-abuse", a euphemism for masturbation. This in turn leads to a wasted and dissolute life.

In a way similar to hiding the Pompeii artefacts, images showing the Cerne Abbas Giant have at times shown him with no penis. No one knows for sure who or what the figure represents, he may be the Roman God Hercules and may have been set in the ground in the reign of the Roman Emperor Commodus between 180 - 193 AD 56. The giant is carved in solid lines from the chalk above the small Dorset village of Cerne Abbas. He is 180 feet high and carries a club which measures 120 feet in length. Apart from the club, his most obvious feature is a huge erect penis.

Local traditions lead some to believe the giant can confer all sorts of benefits, especially regarding fertility but as early as 1774, emasculated images appeared. This is perhaps not surprising as his penis is shown erect and very large. If he is Roman, this would be because the phallus, especially an erect one, was looked upon as a good luck charm. If those viewing the images or the actual hillside figure are of a prudish frame of mind, they will miss what the figure actually represents, it is not pornographic in the modern sense. It is also not erotic, it is not aimed at sexual excitement, rather at increased fertility and good luck in life. Censorship of such artefacts will always be counterproductive because instead of becoming an everyday item, the hidden aspects will give rise to increased interest.

In complete contrast, today we see some images as "high art" that may well have been the pornography of the day. Paintings such as The Martyrdom of Saint Agatha by Sebastiano Del Piombo (ca. 1485-1547) show a woman having her breasts torn off. The painting was commissioned for display in church. The painting Venus, Cupid, Folly and Time by Agnolo Bronzino, circa 1545 hangs in the National Gallery, London. It was commissioned by the Duke of Florence, Cosimo de' Medici as a gift to Francis I of France. The two central figures, Venus and Cupid are both nude Cupid fondles his mother's bare breast and kisses her lips. They are being showered with rose petals by a boy, believed to represent Folly. It appealed to the tastes prevalent both the Medici banking family and the French courts of the time.

If the same scene were painted or photographed today, it would be seen as pornography but because it was painted by a famous a very skilled artist, it has been elevated to the status of high art. Pornography is more in the eye and intention of the viewer than the artist.

What has this to do with naturism? Nudity is not specifically sexual but owing to the confusion in some people's minds over meanings of words, nudity and especially images of nudity, is pornographic. It is my contention that pornography and naturism are poles apart in their motives, porn celebrates excitement without emotion whereas naturism celebrates humans for what they are.

Coming out

Many find that hiding their interest in naturism is the route to an easy life, some even think they are the only ones who enjoy being naked, so tell no-one for fear of being thought eccentric. Fears about coming out are concerned with being ostracised by family and friends, being laughed at or being seen as someone quite odd. As I worked in education, I also feared excessive interest from a possibly conservative employer. For many years, I kept my thoughts to myself and my immediate family. We had enjoyed nude beaches and even time at Le Cap d'Agde, the large naturist town in the South of France, but no-one else knew. After a fairly dramatic change in life occurred, I decided to go the whole way and stop being secretive. Having done so has made a large improvement in my life, "living a lie" is no good to anyone.

Bringing up the subject is not easy, you cannot just come out with it, it must come about in context. When it did, the fear I had felt all those years was found to be baseless, I did not encounter any of the reactions I had been apprehensive about.

The best example is an email I received from a new friend. My wife Rhonda met Penny at a writing course. Penny has trained as a life coach and is interested in encouraging people to achieve their full potential. Rhonda had mentioned that she had had an article published in H&E Naturist magazine so I decided to give Penny the web address of my naturist web site that contains a précis of this book. In her reply she said:

Dear Howard

This is all very fascinating. The article was brilliant. I really admire you for coming out and being true to what you believe. So many people hide their true potential in so many ways thinking others will judge them when they could be really inspirational to others. What you have done is quite symbolic for everyone to live their true lives in whatever way they choose providing they are not harming anyone else in the process.

Saint Francis de Sales wrote:

Do not wish to be anything but what you are, and try and be that perfectly.

Everyone deserves that and to be loved and admired for having the courage to be authentic.

Love from Penny

Could one wish for a better response?

Another friend said to Rhonda, *"I wish I had a husband like yours, it saves on the washing"*. She may not wish to live a naturist lifestyle but this is not the bad reaction so feared for so long.

Much has been made in the past about homosexual people "coming out". In many ways, I have been through the same experience, speaking to friends, neighbours and acquaintances about my life style. Like many before, I have found to my surprise no bad reactions. Most people are encouraging although some are a little bemused. Overall the experience of coming out has lifted a huge burden, the burden of secrecy. Encouraged by my wife's naturist friendly body attitude, all along I have been supported by my close family.

It is easy to conform, to run one's life modelled on those around you. No one bothers you, you do what is expected, life goes on. It takes an effort of will to follow what you believe in, if that belief runs contrary to the norm. Many others have found this down the centuries, they have suffered hate and persecution, those who did not desist or run away were hunted down, imprisoned, tortured or killed. Whilst I am not suggesting that a lifestyle as gentle as naturism results in passions as keenly felt, I do feel the principle holds true, each of us must stand up for what we believe even in the face of opposition. I hold my beliefs in the value of social nudity as strongly as others hold their religious or political beliefs.

If you find that hard to believe or understand, this book is for you.

It will at the very least, outline some of the issues and misconceptions that surround a social nude lifestyle. It is not my aim to promote an outdated view of naturism nor to attempt to recall the days when back to nature was the aim as in the Boulting Brother's film called I'm Alright Jack. [61] It is my intention to say unequivocally, social nudity is enjoyable, harmless and can lead to a much happier life.

> *"We can shed our clothing more easily than we can peel away the psychological effects of civilisation. Undressing takes but a few moments; truly returning to our natural state - if by that we mean releasing ourselves from all post-tribal cultural conditioning - could take a lifetime, at least for adults. And nothing short of amnesia could truly strip us of all that social imprinting, the invisible received assumptions we wear even when naked with our lovers or alone in the bathtub."* [57] *A. D. Coleman*

With friends and strangers

Having "come out", there remains the problem of what to do when others come to my home.

If it is a warm day, should I dress? Having discussed this with a number of friends, it is clear that some are happy if I stay nude, so I do. Others would not be happy, so I dress. The key is to be open and honest about the issue and to ask, not necessarily directly, but to determine how people feel. The same applies with my neighbours, if I am nude in the garden, should I make excessive efforts to remain unseen or should simple discretion. They have the right to live their lives undisturbed, but so do I.

I have summarised some of the problems as a set of possible reactions below:

A friend arrives at the front door who knows about my naturism but has not seen me nude.

Reaction	For	Against
Stay nude	*My desire to lead my own life satisfied*	*Friend may feel uncomfortable even if they say it is ok.*
Put shorts on	*Friend is very likely to feel comfortable and that I have acted to save their embarrassment*	*My desire to lead my own life is compromised*

A friend arrives at the front door who does not know about my naturism.

Reaction	For	Against
Stay nude	*My desire to lead my own life satisfied*	*Friend very likely to be shocked*
Put shorts on	*Friend is very likely to think either I have just been in the bath or that I only wear shorts*	*My desire to lead my own life is compromised*

A stranger arrives at the front door.

Reaction	For	Against
Stay nude	*My desire to lead my own life satisfied*	*Person may be alarmed*
Put shorts on	*Stranger is unaware of the situation*	*My desire to lead my own life is compromised*

A stranger climbs the fence and sees into my private garden.

Reaction	For	Against
Stay nude	*My desire to lead my own life satisfied*	*Person may be alarmed, amused or dismayed*
Put shorts on	*Stranger assumes I feel guitly so must be "up to something"*	*My desire to lead my own life is compromised*

I do the gardening nude.

Reaction	For	Against
Stay nude	*My desire to lead my own life satisfied*	*Neighbours may feel uncomfortable. Even if they are not, their visitors may be.*
Put shorts on	*Neighbours may be pleased*	*My desire to lead my own life is compromised*

In all these cases, most naturists will compromise their lifestyle for the sake of others. Perhaps these others should consider this aspect of society and give more freedom of expression to those around them.

Years of up-bringing are not easy to overcome. The intellectual acceptance of nudity is one thing, emotional acceptance is harder.

Activities

What can you do nude? Anything that does not require protective clothing. Whilst many stay nude around the house in their daily life, the best activities include almost all sports but especially swimming, walking, cycling, golf, boules (petanque) and tennis. It is said that the children's author, Enid Blyton liked to play tennis whilst nude. A form of tennis found only in naturist clubs is called miniten.

A brief search for naturist activities showed that people were doing: Archery, Boating, Boules (Petanque), Building, bungee jumping, Cycling, Dancing, Dining, Golf, Kite Flying, Massage, Miniten, Photography, Reading, Running, Sailing, Sauna, Skiing, Skydiving, Sub aqua diving, Sunbathing, Swimming, Tennis, Tennis, Travel, Volleyball, Walking and Yoga.

There are dozens of nude swims held at local authority swimming pools in the UK and a few local cinemas where guests are not required to dress. People do the gardening and an increasing number have described how they drive nude. Even Noel Edmonds said *"Sometimes I drive it like this with no clothes on and that's really fabulous!"*. The long running and very popular radio programme Gardeners' Question Time featured naturists from Naturist Foundation in Orpington, Kent. It was first broadcast on Sunday 12 July 1998 and the programme was taken as seriously as any other.

There are nude cruises using normal cruise ships and a large number of companies offering nude sailing. The World Naked Bike Ride [58] (WNBR) is organised by many different groups and takes place in cities around the world. Participants are campaigning for a more positive body image.

In addition, many naturists find their religious life is enhanced if they can attend worship nude. Quite a few have got married nude, sometimes where the celebrant I also nude.

Apart from obvious activities where physical protection is required, nudity is not a bar to an active live. Try it!

The official view

Censorship

Anthony Comstock (1844-1915) was a zealous campaigner for censorship in the USA. In 1905, Comstock denounced George Bernard Shaw as an "Irish smut dealer". Shaw retaliated by coining the term "Comstockery". According to Shaw, *"Comstockery is the world's standing joke at the expense of the United States. Europe likes to hear of such things. It confirms the deep-seated conviction of the Old World that America is a provincial place, a second-rate country-town civilisation after all."* It is interesting to note that Shaw could be considered an early naturist. The naturist movement was started in Germany but the ideas of natural living and openness spread to intellectuals such as Shaw. He and his friends would think nothing of a naked bathe in the river.

The situation over in the USA is still the same, it is a society where the Comstock Laws are still in place, a country where a woman's breast is fuzzed out electronically on a television travel program but where extreme violence is portrayed in great detail. Such violence is even celebrated, enormous efforts are used to keep the right to own a gun. In more educated countries where attitudes to humanity are better developed, this situation is reversed. It is common to see women go topless on European beaches, very rare in the USA. Gun crime in the USA has reached epidemic proportions, even in schools, whereas such things are almost unheard of in Europe apart from battles between the drug gangs. The connection between violence and naturism may not be obvious to all, but it is to me. One society values the "me first, make money" attitude, I value the openness and warmth of human society. Naturism encourages openness and the acceptance of others.

Censorship is rife in the USA, even without the support of legislation. Explicit violence is fine, but one must not show various parts of real, un-harmed human bodies. It seems the idea is widespread that a child seeing images of a dead Palestinian on the ground with his blood flowing down the street is less harmful than seeing a naked woman.

I would argue strongly against all centralised and especially governmental censorship. Governments have a different agenda from the rest of society, they wish to stay in power. Any image or text that may tarnish their image is a potential target for their censorship. In the early 20th century, filmed scenes of unemployment were routinely censored, the government did not want the people to know the true state of the economy. The problem is that when a work is cut or banned, one does not get a chance to see the work of the censor, i.e. what was cut. No government can resist the temptation to doctor the news for very long, all have been found wanting in this respect. They will use various excuses for censorship but their real motives are far from honest.

Some politicians will argue for an open, free and democratic society but then pass laws that protect their own brand of religious bigotry. Such people cannot be trusted to censor any media.

One point often missed when discussing censorship, is the choice of people to actually carry out the work. If potential censors feel that harmful or unacceptable material will be presented to them, why have they volunteered to spend much of their working lives watching or listening to it? Is this an act of altruism or do they have darker motives, the desire to watch such material but to disallow others the right to make their own judgement? Why would one apply to do such a job? In the past, censorship has been championed and carried out by people such as Comstock in the USA and Mary Whitehouse in England, people driven by their own religious beliefs. It is their desire to further their religion that drives them on. If you believe in a society where any belief is valued, all religions free to preach their views alongside those who choose not to follow a religious life, then censorship must be bad.

England's version of Comstock was Thomas Bowdler. He is best known for his Family Shakespeare a version where all passages were deleted that *"Cannot with propriety be read aloud in a family"*. Even during his life he was attacked for his prudery, few could understand why literature as great as that of Shakespeare should be the target of such a narrow minded person. He also modified the Old Testament, removing sections *"of an irreligious or immoral tendency"*. As some believe the bible to be the word of God, this showed a breath-taking arrogance. He also bowdlerised Gibbon's History of the Decline and Fall of the Roman Empire, the new verb to bowdlerise is still in use to describe extreme prudery with regard to the arts.

Crime, Politics and the Law

"There is no nonsense so arrant that it cannot be made the creed of the vast majority by adequate government action." Bertrand Russell, *"An Outline of Intellectual Rubbish"*

There is a huge variation in what people call "crime". To make this point, I would like to present two examples that are not directly related to nudity.

1. During the Great War, Winston Churchill sponsored and supported the attack at Gallipoli in 1915. The planning, preparation and execution of the attack and the way it was perpetuated after initial failure, resulted in more than 56,000 allied deaths, 65,000 Turkish deaths and complete loss of prestige for the allied armies and navies. There was no gain whatever. Although after the event he had sufficient integrity to resign, he was not prosecuted. The mistakes made by him and the senior command of the army were so serious and the lack of care taken in the entire campaign so critical to the failure, they have to be considered criminally negligent.

2. When Glenn Stewart landed a Boeing 747 at Heathrow in thick fog, he made a mistake. He was on his own in the flight deck, his first officer was sick and down the back of the aircraft, some of the elderly flight systems were malfunctioning. Under pressure and flying on his own, he made a mistake that resulted in coming too close to a hotel near the airport. After a second attempt, he landed unassisted, no-one was hurt. For having come close to the hotel and having not reported it, he was prosecuted for criminal negligence. At the end of the court case he was found not guilty of endangering an aircraft but guilty of criminal negligence. He then committed suicide.

The point of these examples is to show that the result of normal justice is often at variance with the views of everyday people. One man made a mistake, perhaps he should have diverted to a different airfield with better weather or called for more ground based assistance, but it is hard to understand why he could be found not guilty of endangering an aeroplane but guilty of criminal negligence.

Let me emphasise that again, not just negligence, criminal negligence. In a case such as this, a jury must be told by specialists how aircraft are handled in bad weather, how the two pilots would share the workload of landing in difficult conditions and what role is played by the technical systems, working or not. It is tempting the believe that the jury was told what to think by an establishment keen to show they were on the side of air safety.

What would the outcome have been had Churchill and the senior commanders been tried in 1915? Would this have been a case where technical knowledge would be a key part of a sensible verdict? Churchill sent in the navy first but they failed, this resulted in the Ottoman command being fully prepared for further attacks. Would a jury have been told that insufficient consideration was made of the military problems at Gallipoli, that the high ground behind each beach was a defender's dream? This and other very basic errors were made by the planners. In a court case, it would have been quite clear even to a non-military jury just how incompetent these people had been. Churchill was one of the causes of the pointless deaths of many allied soldiers. Glenn Stewart killed no one apart from himself.

What has this to do with naturism? In the court cases where non sexual public nudity has been the charge, the defendants have been found not guilty of indecency. No technical knowledge or establishment view swayed the jury. They simply took the judgement of 12 of the defendant's peers. In their view, no crime was committed. When viewed by establishment figures, the police, prosecutors etc., public non sexual nudity seems to cause a problem. It suited the establishment to find Glenn Stewart guilty as it showed they were active in flight safety, but it did not suit them to try Churchill as it would have reflected badly on the establishment. It seems there are significant differences between establishment views and those of ordinary people.

Law in the UK

The law in the United Kingdom is not well written when it comes to public nudity, but there is no specific law that prohibits nudity. The original bill drafted for the Sexual Offences Act 2003 contained a clause that caused alarm to naturists, it seemed to imply that nudity itself should attract a two year prison sentence and listing for two years on the sexual offenders register.

That would have effectively ended a person's job prospects for life for what is an innocent act. Life models in art classes would have risked prosecution! After much lobbying by naturists, first the House of Lords and then the Commons amended the bill so that now anyone "exposing his genitals" must be shown to have done so deliberately to cause offence, mere nudity is not an offence. We are assured by the Government that naturists are not affected by this Act. The bill is written using the word "he" but is gender neutral, the act applies to women as well, or at least that is the claim. Physically it is very difficult for a woman to expose her genitals so in writing it, the legislators clearly meant a man. Contrary to any Bill of Human Rights, this legislation makes parts of all men liable to be seen as offensive, i.e. the very fact of being human may be considered illegal. The very same Government passed an ill-considered gun law, its only effect was to end the legitimate sport of pistol shooting. Gun crime has soared. They made the same logical mistake as those who assume naturism is sexual, i.e. *"guns are used in crime, therefore, guns are bad", "sex is often done naked, therefore nakedness is sexual". "Dogs like chocolate, you like chocolate, therefore you are a dog".* Spot the fallacy? It seems the establishment cannot.

Sexual Offences Act 2003

66   Exposure

(1) A person commits an offence if-

(a) he intentionally exposes his genitals, and

(b) he intends that someone will see them and be caused alarm or distress.

(2) A person guilty of an offence under this section is liable-

(a) on summary conviction, to imprisonment for a term not exceeding 6 months or a fine not exceeding the statutory maximum or both;

(b) on conviction on indictment, to imprisonment for a term not exceeding 2 years.

Summary Trial is for minor offences, such as traffic offences and is held at a Magistrates' Court. This court cannot give a custodial sentence more than 6 months or impose fines more than £5000. More serious acts are referred to a Crown Court where Trial on Indictment is held with a jury. The judge is more senior to a Magistrate and may rule on points of law. The jury determines guilt, the judge determines punishment.

Maintenance of control

It means that if we need to control a population, we can choose from several methods. The most obvious is violence, do what I say or you will be hurt or killed. This works in the short term but people placed under such a system eventually rebel so the method is not one of choice for those who wish to retain long term control.

The Romans used violence to achieve their goals but once achieved, they used a more intelligent way to control their conquered lands, reward. Peaceful obedience meant reaping the benefits of prosperity. Of course they had an army as a backstop to quell any violent uprising but the local population enjoyed the advanced systems used by the Romans. Local religions were respected and even incorporated into Roman life. There is plenty of evidence for this, for instance images of local Gods still found in Roman buildings.

Another means to control a population is by religion, do what we say or you will suffer eternal damnation. The problem with this approach is that to work reliably, there must be universal belief, a situation that is difficult to achieve from scratch. A core of true believers can lead by example and hope to demonstrate the benefits of their truth but to achieve a good level of control, a firm grip can only be assured by force, do what we say and you will reap the rewards, fail to do what we say and you will suffer pain on earth and fail to reach paradise.

The Catholic church has made a speciality of this method. The church has used all manner of techniques to further its aims from war to political intrigue, many have been burned at the stake, stoned or tortured to death in the most gruesome manner, all in the name of salvation. What they offer is an interesting mix of benefit and punishment, live the Catholic life and you will live in paradise for ever, disobey the rules and not only will you be cast into hell, you will pay in this life as well.

The next means of controlling a population is by centralising all decision making. Both communist and fascist governments use this, indeed there is not too much difference between them. Individuals are less important than the state so freedoms we take for granted in the West are seen as damaging, they are then rigorously controlled.

All of these methods have force as a final sanction. Individuals have no power and those in power act to stay that way. The idea in a modern democracy is that if force is required, at least it is carried out by trained law officers or the armed services in strictly controlled circumstances and where these people are answerable under the law.

What has this to do with naturism? Naturism is a rational response, if it is hot, don't dress, if it is cold, wrap up. Very few are offended, those that are have been taught to think that way. The legislators need to look closer at why they enact particular laws. It has taken centuries of fighting to achieve democracy and freedom from Church domination so it is unclear why the teachings of a previous system still have such a strong influence. If asked why people conform to a particular mode of behaviour, their answer is likely to that they do it like that because others do it or because it has "always" been done like that, little thinking why.

Campaigners for nudity

As an example of how the police are out of step with common opinion, we need only to consider their actions in response to nude walkers. The following piece was printed in the Guardian newspaper on 6th August 2003. It illustrates just how far the police are from the views of most of the population. A male reporter, Stephen Moss, took part in a nude walk in Epping Forest, a large area of public forest.

"*Now which way back to the car?*"

Stephen Moss dropped everything and struck out into Epping Forest The police, however, are not yet satisfied that boots-(and baguettes-) only hikers pose no threat to the public. "These incidents might be quite tame, but the police are taking them seriously due to the distress they have clearly caused to the public," says acting chief inspector Tadeusz Nowakowski, who is leading the hunt for the intrepid hiker or hikers attempting a naked crossing of the Pennine Way. "Imagine if your wife was stuck up on her own in the dales, having her sandwiches and a bit of a nap, when suddenly this man comes bumbling around the corner."

Clearly the policeman has the 19th Century view where "your wife" is a possession to be protected by the stronger male. Presumably, if a man were to see the nude, all would be well. He seems to think that a women seeing a naked man would be somehow more offended or perhaps feel threatened. He ignores direct evidence to the contrary, nude walkers generally encounter either neutral or positive reactions. When on a nude walk with a group of naturists, one of whom was an ex police officer, I asked how he would decide what to do when reports came in of nude walkers in the local area. He said *"It comes down to individuals"*. Hardly a policy for equitable law enforcement.

At about the same time as Stephen Moss was trying a nude walk, several people were campaigning nude for the Right to be Yourself. One of them, Steven Gough, undertook to walk the length of the country nude. It is walks such as that that are referred to above where the acting Chief Inspector was *"leading the hunt"*. The bad reactions that Steve Gough experienced were from the police, not from the general public, he was arrested and imprisoned under various public order acts. When in prison he refused to wear clothes so was forcibly kept in solitary confinement.

It is hard to understand why the police and courts treated him like this, but the history of Britain has records of many similar events, people being imprisoned and maltreated for their beliefs. He tried the same defence as Vincent Bethel as described below, i.e. to be naked in court before they decided if nudity was bad. When he insisted he remain nude, he was taken below and a lawyer pressed into presenting his case. He was found guilty, thereby creating a clear miscarriage of justice, he was not allowed to speak for himself in court, the case had been decided beforehand.

In the history of this land, eventually right prevails, so I have every confidence that non sexual public nudity will be found to comply with the law, it will just take time for the court officials and the police to catch up with society. When juries consider fairly presented cases of public nudity, they throw them out. When released, Steve Gough resumed and eventually finished his walk, naked.

Some campaigning individuals insist they are not naturists. They make this judgement because they see the naturist establishment in Britain as stuffy and inward looking and have no wish to be associated with them. The establishment is seen as preferring to hide behind the fences of "nudist colonies" that gives the tabloids so much fun in the silly season. In the view of some often high profile campaigners, they campaign to be nude in public as a human right, their campaign is known as *"the right to be yourself"*. Some have been in prison for their beliefs and must be admired for their tenacity.

One, Vincent Bethel, used an interesting defence at his trial. He was arrested and charged after such stunts as climbing naked up a lamp standard outside Buckingham Palace. He did this and other tricks many times with the intention of being arrested so he could pursue in the courts his claim to the right to be nude. When ordered to dress for his court appearance, he refused on the grounds that if he had to be dressed, the court had pre-judged his case.

He insisted that he had the right to be nude unless he was found guilty. The judge recognised his claim was correct, so he was nude in court the whole time, as was at least one witness. The mixed gender jury was asked if they objected, none did. He was acquitted so walked free, and naked, from the court. He had made a strong point, in general, the British do not object to non-sexual nudity, even if they do not choose to join in.

115

In Germany, Austria and other continental countries, there are public parks where nudity is the norm. When non-naturists stroll past naked people, no problem arises. When a naked event was planned in Hyde Park in London in the summer of 2003, the police were told of the date and time and that the event was not a protest, simply a picnic for naked friends. On the day, the police outnumbered the picnickers at least two to one and used unnecessary threats to prevent anyone undressing. One man did undress but felt so intimidated by the police behaviour that he dressed again. It is not easy to understand why continental police should be largely absent from the naturist areas of their city parks but the British police turn up in force.

In Cambridge there is Richard Collins, a campaigning naturist who cycles nude along the public highway. He has been arrested a few times but it does not stop him, it seems now that in this area the police tolerate his lifestyle to some extent, they seem to realise that he presents no threat to anyone.

He has appeared on the radio and television to publicise his activity, he has also informed the police to ensure they know what he intends to do. He does it as part of his campaign for the right to be himself.

The National Trust took an odd attitude to naturists at Studland Bay on the South coast of England. The area has been used without trouble by naturists for many years but one National Trust individual took it into his head to restrict the size of the area being used. The official policy of the NT is one of tolerance, a policy derived from the opinion of ordinary people who sit on their governing body but when it comes to individuals who have been given too much power, minorities often suffer.

There are naturists who insist on being nude whilst washing their car in the front of their house, they claim their neighbours do not mind. Whilst I can understand their wish to feel free and dress sensibly to wash the car, the fact that some neighbours do not complain does not mean they are happy. Too many of the poorer sort of British businesses use this as a measure of customer satisfaction, no complaints equals satisfied customers! Clearly this is not a situation that will lead to common acceptance of naturism, what is required is dialogue and understanding.

Politics

It is said that *"Politics is the art of the possible"*. If that were true, any legislation passed would conform not to common sense but to the political climate at the time. A number of new Acts passed in the UK Parliament and the US Senate have shown this to be untrue, they have been carried by the majority in the house but would not have been passed by a majority in the country. This leads to bad law as people do not respect the new laws and start to choose which law to obey and which not.

Some of the Members of the UK Parliament are naturists themselves but in general do not speak up for the nude lifestyle. This is one aspect of modern political life where image is placed above conviction, where presentation wins over substance.

Lessons should be learned from the experience of others, anyone who ignores history is doomed to repeat it. In the most repressive Western countries, the rates of what religious people would describe as "immoral behaviour" are higher. The USA has some very repressive laws regarding nudity; even where the law itself is written in a reasonable way, the manner in which the police and courts behave results in the same thing, repression. In France where people are much less repressed, the average age at first intercourse is higher for teenagers. The birth-rate, abortion rate, and instances of AIDS are all far lower in the same age group. Compared with Europe, the rate of teenage pregnancy is four times higher in the USA. People do not obey repressive laws, they hide their actions.

The American show Hair had a famous nude scene, but at the time, theatres were censored by the Lord Chamberlain, a member of the Royal Household. His approval was unlikely so the actors for the UK show were placed on retainers until this situation could be resolved. In fact, the problem went away when the Lord Chamberlain lost his task of censoring theatres. The show went on to be seen by large numbers of people.

In 1972 the Oz magazine was prosecuted for "Corrupting Public Morals". An issue of the magazine that had been published in 1970 was used as evidence. The editors were found guilty of the lesser charge of obscenity and sent to jail. There was widespread public anger at a custodial sentence for these people and the case became one of the most celebrated legal cases concerning censorship.

The 20th February 1973 edition of the Sun newspaper included a large photograph of Jilly Johnson nude. It was thought to be quite controversial at the time but it started the "page three girl" image that helped to sell millions of copies of the Sun.

Rosie Boycott started a Women's Liberation magazine called Spare Rib. In the aftermath of the Oz trial and the start of the page three girl editions of the Sun, Cosmopolitan magazine published a series of male nudes as a counter to the increasing number of female nudes; the feminist position taken by Spare Rib and others was that women were being exploited only for their bodies. About one of these male nudes, Rosie Boycott said *"His dangly bits are hidden by the middle of the fold, you can't really see them, but the great thing was, no one cared. It was completely boring. I mean you took a look at it and you giggled. Actually they looked so stupid. There is something interesting about the male nude to the female, you love and like men for something more than their bodies"*.

Political protests and campaigners for peace

In recent times there has been an increase in nudity used as a means to gain publicity for political protest. From a naturist point of view this is not a good development as it underlines the idea that nudity is out of the ordinary. In a more sensible society, nudity would not be an issue so would not work as a means of attracting attention.

Members of Rylstone and District Women's Institute made their now very famous nude calendar to raise funds for Leukaemia Research. It succeeded in raising a huge amount and the whole story was made into the successful film Calendar Girls. Many people jumped on the bandwagon, there are now a very large number of nude calendars, the more there are, the less effective they will become at attracting attention.

Nudity as a tactic was used by the Doukhobors in the early 20th century. Doukhobor is a Russian word that means "Spirit Wrestler", a name applied in the 18th century to a group of people who refused to give up their faith in favour of the Orthodox Church. Following emigration to Canada their problems were not over, their communal living being at odds with the culture of free enterprise and military service seen as essential by Canadians. Following strong government action, a Doukhobor faction called The Sons of Freedom used eccentric forms of protest including marching in the nude.

In the early 21st Century, campaigns such as Naked For Peace [59] have used nudity to gain their desired publicity. The organisation People for the Ethical Treatment of Animals [60] (PETA) have followed suit as have people intent on stopping the running of bulls in Pamplona [61].

Slogans such as these have become common: *"Disrobe for disarmament"*, *"Nudes, not nukes!"*, *"Naked For Peace"*, *"Dare 2 Bare 4 Freedom + Peace"*, *"I'd rather go naked than wear fur!"* and *"I Got Rid Of My Bush! Read My Lips - No To War!"*

As nudity becomes more commonplace, campaigners will need other means to attract attention.

Conclusion

To me naturism greatly improves my life, my happiness. My belief in the rightness of this lifestyle is as genuine as any belief in religious ideals. I recognise that nudity causes some people problems so I am very careful not to offend them, but I also recognise that I have rights to my beliefs, the same way as they have theirs. The solution is not all or nothing, it lies in the good old British compromise. Leave me to lead my naked life and I will do my best not to offend, I will respect your lifestyle and no my best not to be offended by it.

Attitudes to social nudity are improving, at least in Europe. People from the USA are able to take home their experience of this better attitude and will eventually be able to break down the very prudish behaviour of the US law makers and the more extreme elements of the Christian right wing. Naturism can be seen as a better alternative to the enjoyment of violence and the projection of US power by military means, it promotes equality and peace rather than inequality and war. The current love of violence in the USA will only lead to misery for all, no one wins military battles, plenty win attitude battles.

Experiencing a socially nude environment, people find that any embarrassment disappears very quickly. The barrier to social nudity is far harder to overcome from the clothed side. Once the initial unfamiliar feeling has gone, most are left with a strong impression that no real problem ever existed. I would recommend that in the privacy of your own home, take your clothes off and go about your normal routine. It may feel strange for a while, but enjoy the experience, naturists do. You may not feel you need to take the next step, to participate in a naturist swim, a walk in the countryside or a visit a nude beach, but at least you will have come some way to understanding why naturists love being naked. Freedom.

Appendices

About me

For as long as I can remember but certainly as early as the age of six, I have enjoyed being without clothes. No one knew I felt that way but I did not feel it was in any way odd. Not knowing that both my parents had met at a naturist establishment and that nudity was nothing to fear, I kept it very quiet. After all, I was the only person in the world to feel like this. It was only later that I learnt of the existence of "nudist colonies". Sometime during my teens I saw a film called I'm Alright Jack. [62] This film opens in a naturist club and ends with short sequence where a mixed group of naked people are seen running off into the countryside. No sex, just enjoying the sun and air.

This was an enormous revelation to me, it was clear others felt the same way as I did and it was OK, there were even places where people socialised naked. I resolved to find out more. I am still finding out.

Statistics

Canada

A national Survey on Canadian attitudes was published by The Federation of Canadian Naturists in 1999. [64] 51% of recipients of this postal survey resulted in:

• 2.7 million Canadians (8.9% of households) either have visited or are willing to visit clothing-optional locations.

• An additional 3.5 million Canadians (11.6% of households) are "comfortable with skinny-dipping in mixed company."

• 11.8 million Canadians (39% of households) have walked or would walk around their house nude.

United Kingdom

The information below was taken from a survey was commissioned by British Naturism. Much more detail is available in the full report.

The following questions were included in a survey for British Naturism and asked by NOP in their regular "Omnibus" survey. The 1823 people questioned between February 8 and 13, 2001 were from a demographically representative sample of the UK population, aged 16 and over. The results are interesting and are summarised below:

Experience of unclothed activities

Have you ever:

Sunbathed without a costume to get an all-over tan?	*14%*
Swum without a costume?	*24%*
Been on a foreign naturist beach?	*11%*
Visited a British clothes optional beach, resort or club?	*7%*

Attitudes to naturists. Naturists enjoy activities such as sunbathing and swimming without clothes.

Do you think such people are:

Criminal?	*2%*
Disgusting?	*7%*
Harmless?	*88%*
Sensible?	*40%*

Attitudes to encountering nudity.

You are walking along the coast on a hot day, and come across a group of naked people sunbathing, swimming or playing cricket, would you:

Ignore them and keep walking?   *78%*

Be alarmed and keep well away from them?   *2%*

Go naked yourself?   *2%*

Settle down but keep your swimming costume on?   *13%*

Call the police because you were frightened or distressed?   *1%*

Attitudes to public nudity and the law.

If not intended to give offence, do you think adult nudity should be legal

In back gardens?   *66%*

In quiet areas of public parks?   *10%*

At certain times in public swimming pools?   *35%*

Anywhere that is specifically declared a "clothing optional" zone?   *69%*

Would you describe yourself as a naturist or not?

Yes   *2%*

No   *97%*

Refused   *1%*

Don't know   *1%*

NB. in the above surveys, an answer such as "not since I was a child" counts as "no". An answer such as "only on my own" counts as "yes".

USA

In 1983, Gallop Organisation carried out a poll [63] commissioned by The Naturist Society. The people of the Naturist Education Foundation thought that by the year 2000, the 1983 results would not reflect the current attitudes so they re-ran the poll. The results are shown side by side below.

	1983		*2000*	
	Yes	No	Yes	No
Do you believe that people who enjoy nude sunbathing should be able to do so without interference from officials as long as they do so at a beach that is accepted for that purpose?	72	24	80	17
Local and state governments now set aside public land for special types of recreation such as snow-mobiling, surfing and hunting. Do you think special and secluded areas should be set aside for people who enjoy nude sunbathing	39	54	48	48
Have you, personally, ever gone "skinny dipping" or nude sunbathing in a mixed group of men and women at a beach, at a pool, or somewhere else?	15	83	25	73

The 2000 Poll shows that one of every four adults in the U.S. has at least experimented in a socially nude environment. With the current population of the US, this extrapolates to an estimated 51 million people.

References

1   Robert Tedder, http://www.personal.u-
    net.com/~tedder/nats/denial.htm
2   Writings of Alfred North Whitehead, British mathematician, logician
    and philosopher
3   Professor Mark Williams, http://www.nhs.uk/conditions/stress-
    anxiety-depression/pages/mindfulness.aspx
4   Caroline Walker, British Naturism BN161, Autumn 2004
5   1999 National Survey on Canadian Attitudes Towards Nudity,
    http://www.fcn.ca/survey.html
6   Survey of opinion towards nudity in the USA,
    http://www.nef.oshkosh.net/Projects/NEF-Roper_Poll/nef-
    roper_poll.html
7   The Human Race. T. Dixon and M. Lucas. Book Club Associates
8   Clothes, Clay and Beauty care,
    http://www.andaman.org/book/chapter13/text13.htm
9   http://www.tigressproductions.co.uk/profile/jb.html
10 Desmond Morris. The Human Animal, BBC Books, ISBN 0563
    370211
11 E. L. Kirchner, Diary 1923
12 USA Today (Magazine), March, 1998 by Anthony Layng
    http://www.findarticles.com/p/articles/mi_m1272/is_n2634_v126/ai_
    20409128
13 http://www.tekline.co.uk/natusa.htm
14 Nikki Craft, Nudist Hall of Shame,
    http://www.nostatusquo.com/ACLU/NudistHallofShame
15 Hermann Goering, Commander-in-Chief of the Luftwaffe, Born
    1893, Suicide 1946.
    http://perso.wanadoo.fr/normand/nateur/fr/site.htm
16 W. Will van der. The Transition of German Culture to National
    Socialism . http://www.history-of-the-
    holocaust.org/LIBARC/LIBRARY/Themes/State/Will.html
17 Shane Steinkamp
    http://www.theplacewithnoname.com/library/nud/p/selfloathing.htm
18 Oxford English Dictionary.
19 Richard Dawkins, The Selfish Gene, Oxford University Press,
    October 1989, ISBN: 0192860925

20 *The Evolution of Meme Machines, Conference Paper delivered at the International Congress on Ontopsychology and Memetics, Milan (18-21 May 2002), Dr. Susan Blackmore.*
    http://intraspec.ca/meme.php

21 *NOP for British Naturism, February 8 and 13, 2001*

22 *Angelius Silesius (1624-1677), German poet also known as Johann Scheffler*

23 *http://www.literature.org/authors/darwin-charles/the-voyage-of-the-beagle/chapter-08.html*

24 *http://www.literature.org/authors/darwin-charles/the-voyage-of-the-beagle/chapter-05.html*

25 *Bill Bryson, Mother Tongue,. Penguin Books. ISBN 014014305X*

26 *Ruling Passions. Shown on BBC2, March 1995. 6-part documentary series, co-production with Roger Bolton Productions Limited.*

27 *Peter Matthiessen*

28 *Dorothy Rowe, The Successful Self. Fontana Paperbacks. ISBN: 0-00-637342-9*

29 *Edward DeBono, I am Right, You are Wrong, Penguin Books, ISBN 0140126783*

30 *Ignatius of Loyola, Founder of the Society of Jesus, known as the Jesuits*

31 *L.P. (Leslie Poles) Hartley (1895-1972), British author. The Go-Between, prologue (1953).*

32 *British Museum Little Book of Erotica, Catherine Johns, IBN 0-7141-5026-0*

33 *British Museum accession number EA 10008/3*

34 *British Museum accession number GR 1999.4-26.1*

35 *British Museum accession number OA 1964.4-13.1*

36 *deHoratev, op. cit.*

37 *Karen Armstrong. A History of God. Vintage Books, London, 1999, ISBN 0-7493-0692-0*

38 *Speech at the International Union for Conservation of Nature and Natural Resources general assembly in New Delhi, India, 1968*

39 *Thomas Fuller*

40 *Florence Dupont, Christopher Woodall, Daily Life in Ancient Rome, Blackwell ISBN: 0631193952*

41 *Clement of Alexandria, The Educator Book III, Chapter X.-The Exercises Suited to a Good Life*

42 Mikkel Aaland, Mass Bathing: The Roman Bainea and Thermae. 1997

43 Roy Bowen Ward, Women in Roman Baths, Harvard Theological Review 85:2, 1992).

44 Jacques Ellul. Professor at the University of Bordeaux, 1912-1944

45 Reay Tannahill, Sex in History, 1992, ISBN 0812885406

46 Augustine c. duas epist, Pelag. I 34, 17

47 St. Augustine, Treatise on the Correction of the Donatists (417)

48 Pictura in Cappella Ap.ca coopriantur.

49 Cristo della Minerva, Church of Santa Maria sopra Minerva, Rome

50 Nigel Davies, The Rampant God: Eros Throughout the World, 1984, ISBN 0688030947

51 Published Psychology Summary. http://www.geocities.com/yolonz/nfn/psych_summary.htm

52 Werner Zimmermann. Liebesklarheit. Eine Frucht aus Erlebnis, Erkenntnis und Tat (1927)

53 http://www.guardian.co.uk/

54 Channel 4, (11 October 2001) The Secret History of Civilisation - Pornography.

55 Pornography: The Secret History of Civilisation , Isabel Tang ISBN: 0752217925

56 http://www.mysteriousbritain.co.uk/majorsites/cerne_abbass.html

57 A. D. Coleman, Introduction in Naked In Paradise, Michael von Graffenried. Dewi Lewis Publishing, ISBN 189923585X

58 http://www.worldnakedbikeride.org/

59 http://www.sfheart.com/naked_for_peace.html

60 http://www.peta.org

61 http://www.runningofthenudes.com

62 I'm Alright Jack. Film by Boulting Brothers, 1959

63 http://www.nef.oshkosh.net/Projects/NEF-Roper_Poll/nef-roper_poll.html

64 http://www.fcn.ca/survey.html

65 Pioneer plaque courtesy NASA/JPL-Caltech https://commons.wikimedia.org/wiki/File:Pioneer_plaque.svg

Also available:

Naked Hiking by Richard Foley

Naturist Red in Tooth and Claw by Stuart Pitsligo

One, Two, Free! by Anita and Wolfgang Gramer

Promoted Beyond Glory (series) by Stuart Pitsligo

The World Naked Bike Ride by Richard Foley

Romance Scam by Brigitte Schmid

for these and other interesting books connect with us online:

http://pub.rfi.net